高等医学院校教材

外科基本操作导论
（双语版）

主　编　汤文浩　刘志勇

东 南 大 学 出 版 社
·南京·

内 容 提 要

外科基本操作是每位临床医学专业学生的必修课。本教材是按 48 学时(12 次实验,每次 4 学时)编写的一本外科基本操作指导性教材,内容包括无菌术、外科基本操作(切开、止血、结扎、缝合)、腹腔镜基本操作、创伤急救基本技术、心肺复苏基本技术和动物模拟手术训练等。

本书可以作为医学院各专业的医学生学习外科基本操作的指导教材。

图书在版编目(CIP)数据

外科基本操作导论 / 汤文浩,刘志勇主编. —南京:
东南大学出版社,2013.1(2022.1 重印)
汉英双语教材
ISBN 978-7-5641-4065-6

Ⅰ.①外… Ⅱ.①汤… ②刘… Ⅲ.①外科手术—操
作—双语教学—高等学校—教材 Ⅳ.①R615

中国版本图书馆 CIP 数据核字(2012)第 318790 号

外科基本操作导论

出版发行:东南大学出版社
社　　址:南京市四牌楼 2 号　邮编:210096
出 版 人:江建中
责任编辑:戴坚敏
网　　址:http://www.seupress.com
电子邮箱:press@seupress.com
经　　销:全国各地新华书店
印　　刷:广东虎彩云印刷有限公司
开　　本:787mm×1092mm　1/16
印　　张:12.5
字　　数:326 千字
版　　次:2013 年 1 月第 1 版
印　　次:2022 年 1 月第 4 次印刷
书　　号:ISBN 978-7-5641-4065-6
定　　价:45.00 元

Introduction to Basic Surgical Skills
Bilingual Edition
（A Guide Book for Undergraduate Surgical Education）

Edited by

Wen-hao Tang，M. D.，Ph. D.
Professor of Surgery
Department of General Surgery
School of Medicine
Southeast University

Zhi-yong Liu，M. D.
Professor of Surgery
Department of Cardiothoracic Surgery
School of Medicine
Southeast University

编写人员

柏志斌　　　东南大学医学院血管外科　　　　　　　　　讲　师
（实习四）

蒋小华　　　东南大学医学院普外科　　　　　　　　　　副教授
（实习二、三）

李俊生　　　东南大学医学院普外科　　　　　　　　　　副教授
（实习八）

刘志勇　　　东南大学医学院心胸外科　　　　　　　　　教　授
（实习九、十、十二）

秦永林　　　东南大学医学院血管外科　　　　　　　　　副教授
（实习五）

石　欣　　　扬州大学医学院附属苏北人民医院普外科　　副教授
（实习六）

汤文浩　　　东南大学医学院普外科　　　　　　　　　　教　授
（概述、实习一）

尤承忠　　　东南大学医学院普外科　　　　　　　　　　讲　师
（附录）

CONTRIBUTORS

Zhi-bin Bai, M. D. , Ph. D.
Lecturerof Surgery
Department of Vascular Surgery
School of Medicine
Southeast University
(Session 4)

Xiao-hua Jiang, M. D. , Ph. D.
Associate Professor of Surgery
Department of General Surgery
School of Medicine
Southeast University
(Session 2 and Session 3)

Jun-sheng Li, M. D. , Ph. D.
Associate Professor of Surgery
Department of General Surgery
School of Medicine
Southeast University
(Session 8)

Zhi-yong Liu, M. D. , Ph. D.
Professor of Surgery
Department of Cardiothoracic Surgery
School of Medicine
Southeast University
(Session 9, Session 10 and Session 12)

Yong-lin Qin, M. D. , Ph. D.
Associate Professor of Surgery
Department of Vascular Surgery
School of Medicine
Southeast University
(Session 5)

Xin Shi, M. D. , Ph. D.
Associate Professor of Surgery
Department of General Surgery
Affiliated Subei People's Hospital
School of Medicine
Yangzhou University
(Session 6)

Wen-hao Tang, M. D. , Ph. D.
Professor of Surgery
Department of General Surgery
School of Medicine
Southeast University
(Course Overview and Session 1)

Cheng-zhong You, M. D. , Ph. D.
Lecturer of Surgery
Department of General Surgery
School of Medicine
Southeast University
(Appendix)

前　言

　　飞行员在驾驶飞机离地之前就可以有娴熟的飞行技能,他们是通过高仿真飞行模拟器获得这些技能的。在外科学习曲线的初期阶段,我们也可以采用类似的模拟训练方法。本书的目的就是为初学者创立一个外科技能训练课程,使医学生在进入手术室之前就能掌握一些基本手术技能,缩短在真实病人身上的学习曲线,减少不必要的手术技巧方面的并发症,缩短手术用时。本课程的训练包括桌面实验、盒式训练器和动物实验等。

　　为了培养正确、精细的外科操作技术,我国医学院在课程设置中已经将外科基本操作归入必修课,并且纳入评估体系。该课程一般在医学院的三年级开课,旨在按课程设置要求介绍外科基本操作技巧,要求学生通过外科手术基本操作的强化训练,打好外科手术操作的基础。实践证明,许多外科技巧可以在外科实验室内讲授,医学生可以通过用动物器官或用活体动物进行外科技术训练,并结合计算机辅助教学及视频,提高手术技能。

　　手术是一种团队工作。本课程要求学生以小组(通常 4～5 人为一组)为单位,进行强化动手操作训练。在我国医学院校中,该课程的教学内容主要包括无菌术、外科基本操作技术和心肺复苏基本技术三方面。尽管外科无菌技术和手术基本操作的基本原则相同,但具体方法各院校仍有差异。为了履行以能力为导向的外科技能培养方案,本书列出了 5 种动物模拟手术操作,目的是让每个学生都有操作机会。结合我院具体情况,我们作了适当调整。在 5 次手术中,安排了 2 次小肠部分切除端—端吻合术,旨在将无菌技术与手术操作相结合,要求学生在执行无菌技术的前提下,对外科手术基本操作(切开、分离、止血、结扎、缝合)有多练的机会,从而打好外科操作的基础。

汤文浩　刘志勇

2012 年重阳节于南京丁家桥 87 号

PREFACE

Airline pilots become proficient at flying an aeroplane before even leaving the ground, acquiring skills on a high-fidelity flight simulator. The analogous situation should be possible for the early part of the learning curve in surgery. The aim of this booklet was to develop a beginner-based surgical skill training program for the initial acquisition of technical skill, leading to a basic level of proficiency prior to entering the operating theater and reducing their learning curve on real patients. This may lead to a reduction in the number of unnecessary complications occurring due to a failure of technical skills, and the time spent in the operating room. Basic and procedural tasks can be simulated in a bench, box trainer or animal model environment.

In order to provide training on correct, delicate and precise surgical techniques, the basic surgical skill training course is integrated in the Medical Curriculum as a mandatory requirement for the students major in clinical medicine in China. This training course is usually undertaken within the 3rd academic year of medical students in University, offers an introduction to fundamental surgical skills required by Medical Curriculum and focuses on training students to acquire a higher level of basic skills in open surgery by means of intense laboratory practice. Evidence shows that many surgical skills can be taught in the environment of a surgical skills laboratory. Medical students can develop and improve their surgical skills by participating in workshops that combine the use of animal organs, live animals, computer-aided learning programs and videotapes.

Surgery is a team work. The emphasis of this course is on small group (usually 4 to 5 students) working, intensive hands-on practice of basic skills and the performance of practical procedures. Although there are minor variations in the way that basic surgical skills are taught to medical students at medical schools in China, three modules are undertaken over the forty-eight hours of the course: surgical aseptic techniques, basic surgical skills in open surgery and basic skills in cardiopulmonary resuscitation, especially for trauma patients. To implement a competency-based surgical skills curriculum, training of basic surgical skills was considered an important learning goal in the operative field. Thus, in our school, repeating Session 10 twice was integrated with focus on enhancing basic suturing techniques on animal models, although four different hands-on training programs on animal models have been offered in this book.

Wen-hao Tang
Zhi-yong Liu

目　　录

CONTENTS

Course Overview

Surgery treats illness by manual or operative methods. Although there is quite a different kind of surgeries involved in a variety of surgical specialties, there are common basic aseptic rules and surgical elements such as instrument-handlings, incision, exposure, dissection, hemostasis, ligation (knot tying) and suture, which will be implemented and studied using examples from different subject matters such as the use of nonsynthetic materials and animals. The ethos of the Basic Surgical Skills course is to install core surgical skills and develop aseptic methods at the very beginning of a surgeon's training by teaching the correct basic technique.

The surgical skills training and education laboratory is a state-of-the-art educational facility that provides an environment to teach fundamental technical skills and procedures, where students can learn and hone their technical skills prior to performing procedures on a real patient.

Students entering the Surgical Skill Lab should rigorously adhere to the same principles of asepsis as surgeon entering the human operating room (OR), which is the foundation of surgical site infection prevention. Pay serious attention to all the steps in the practice, provide care for animals (humaneness for the animals) and prevent animal from anesthetic accident, surgical site infection and accidental death.

A. INSTRUCTION FOR STUDENTS ENTERING THE SURGICAL SKILL LAB

1. People dressed in street clothes or clothes worn elsewhere about the campus are not appreciated to enter the Surgical Skill Lab and a clean white smock or coat is recommended.

2. You must change into clogs or sandals at the barrier between the Lab and the rest of the campus.

3. Before entering the Lab, you need to enter the changing room, where you should put on a cap/hood and make sure it completely covers your hair, the scalp line and sideburn (Fig. 0-1). A face mask must be up over the nose, if it fogs your glasses, arrange its top edge, so that your breath does not drift upwards, or, rub your glasses with ordinary soap and polish them. Then you must change into a scrub suit, consisting of pants and a short sleeved shirt. The shirt is tucked inside the trousers, not allowed to hang loosely

(Fig. 0-2). Underwear should be made of cotton. Other material such as silk，wool，nylon，dacron，orlon，and rayon can carry a highelectric charge. A spark from these can be very dangerous in the presence of the highly inflammable anesthetic gases. A clean scrub suit is donned whenever personnel enter the restricted or semirestricted area of the operating room.

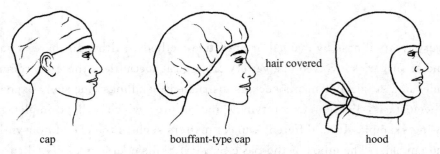

cap   bouffant-type cap   hair covered   hood

Fig. 0-1　Hair cover types
图 0-1　戴帽遮发

4. Be serious in the practice and follow teacher (program directors)'s instruction. Talking is kept to a minimum during surgery. No loud talking, no laughing, no shouting or crying out.

5. Surgery is a collaborative effort. Each member of the team has specific duties and tasks that complement the other members and achieve common goals.

6. Surgery requires extreme concentration and a high sense of responsibilities. Although it is a skill training course on animal models, carelessness or perfunctoriness is not accepted.

7. When the surgery is completed, soiled instruments should be cleaned, washed, disinfected, dried, lubricated, packaged and then taken to the sterilization room.

8. Before leaving the operating room after an infected case, personnel should put gloves, caps, masks and gowns in the containers provided specifically for this purpose. Soiled scrub suits must be placed in a marked laundry receptacle so that they do not spread contamination.

9. Practice strict economy，keep the operative environment clean and tidy，take good care of surgical instruments，equipments and furniture.

10. A perfect knot tying requiring a great deal of practice, each student will practice the knot tying by means of several homework assignments. Take your time when learning

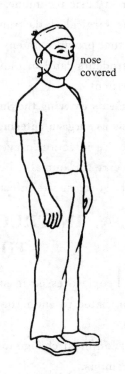

nose covered

Fig. 0-2　OR（operating room）attire
图 0-2　手术室的着装

these skills. It is better to be methodical and slow at first. Speed and efficiency will follow with practice if you use the same technique repeatedly. After each session of hands-on training on animal models, students are expected to write lab protocols: making anesthesia note by anesthetist and dictating operative and postoperative reports by surgeons, referring to Appendix 3. Certification of successful completion is based on following skills assessments: knot tying, aseptic techniques (scrubbing, gloving and gowning), cardio-pulmonary resuscitation and medical records writing.

B. OPERATING ROOM PERSONNEL

Each member of the team has a clearly assigned role and responsibility. Students will work in small groups preparing and operating on animals, but they are encouraged to work in a cooperative way to complete performance objectives, demonstrating integrity and holistic view.

1. Surgeon (operator) usually stands on the right side of patients (Fig. 0-3) and is responsible for operation, including incision, dissection, homeostasis, ligature and suture, under the prescribed policies or according to intraoperative events, directs the surgical team during the procedure.

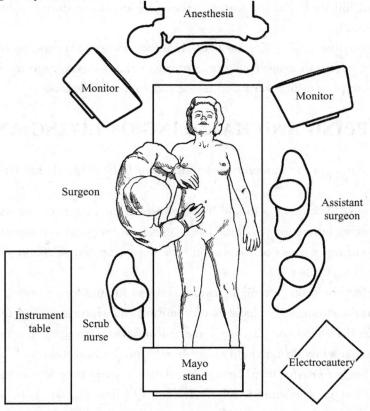

Fig. 0-3 Positioning of the sterile team members and the furniture
图 0-3 手术组人员和设施的位置

2. The first assistant, scrubbing ahead of operator, may perform surgical skin preparation, works with scrubbed nurse to unfold the drapes over patient, stands on opposite side to surgeon and is responsible for hemostasis and sucking blood during the procedure.

3. The second assistant, standing by the operator or the first assistant, is responsible for holding retractors, cutting thread and sucking blood.

4. Scrubbed nurse scrubs before the rest of the sterile team to prepare all sterile supplies and equipment that have been previously opened. Scrub nurse, usually standing adjacent to the operator at about the level of the thighs, is responsible for instruments and it delivery, needle-threading, sutures, devices, solutions, and medications according to the specific surgery, maintaining a clean and orderly managed instrument table and sterile field, protecting the surgical setup from contamination, and performing the initial instrument, sponge, and needle count with the circulator.

All items that could be retained in the surgical wound are counted by two people in a prescribed manner. Policies directing sponge, sharps, and instrument counts (called simply a count) have been established. The count is performed before surgery begins to establish a baseline count, before closure of a cavity, and before skin closure.

5. Anesthetist: Anesthetist is responsible for anesthesia, meticulous assessment, monitoring, and adjustment of the patient's physiological status during surgery. Stands on the head of the table.

6. The circulating nurse: The tasks of circulator were as follows: to fetch and carry, to place the kick bucket or other sponge receptacle in close proximity to the sterile field, to participate in count, to secure scrubbed nurse and surgeons' gowns.

C. TRAPPING AND HANDLING OF LIVING ANIMALS

Dogs or rabbits are the common used animals for basic surgical skill training in Southeast University.

1. If it is possible, animals should be purchased from a supplier and moved to the cages or kennel of experimental lab one week ahead of the studies, especially for dogs, which serves to bridge periods of adaptation to new environments, thereby reducing stress and experimental variability.

2. Except for drinking, overnight fasting allows 12 hours for emptying of the stomach before the operation to minimize hazards of vomiting and aspiration, and to help exposure and operation in the abdomen. These are the reasons why fasting is appropriate for a dog or cat, but these reasons do not hold true for rabbits, because rabbits lack the vomiting reflex and can begin to suffer liver damage in relatively short time when the gut is empty, although rabbit gut passage time is relatively long (12 hours). So, it is not advisable to fast the rabbit before surgery.

3. Catching and restraint of animal

（1）Dog capture is more difficult and chemical immobilization with ketamine/acepromazine is normally used. The drug is injected by hand with a syringe into the rear leg muscles after the dog was confined with the help of a squeeze cage, or restrained by a special catch loop. An intractable dog may need to be muzzled. A muzzle must be fitted snugly so that it protects against bites, but at the same time it must be comfortable for the dog. A commercial muzzle may be purchased in many sizes, or a gauze muzzle may used as described below (Fig. 0-4).

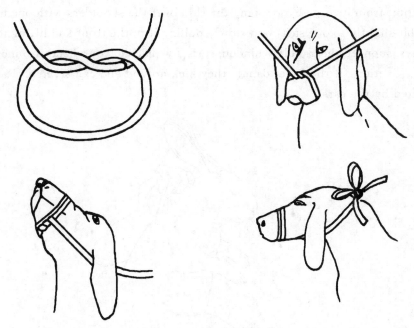

Fig. 0-4　The way to make a temporary muzzle
图 0-4　狗鼻口的捆缚方法

First, take a cotton tape approximately 100 cm in length and 1~1.5 cm in width and make a large loop with a loose knot in a single throw. A large loop allows you to keep your hands at a safe distance until the muzzle is tied. Slowly and gently, slip it over the dog's jaws. Secure the knot on top of his nose, and then tie another loop with a single-throw knot below the mouth. Finally, tie it behind the head, with a bow. **Although all knots must be secured, the muzzle should not be so tight anywhere as to pinch the skin.** This would be painful and would cause the dog to struggle.

To remove the muzzle, untie it at the back, and again keeping your hands away from the dog, slowly pull the gauze strip towards you. Note how the steady, gentle pull loosened the knots around his jaws without hurting him. That is why only single-throw knots should be used.

A muzzle should be removed immediately if a dog has difficulty breathing or starts to vomit.

（2）Rabbits need to be handled very carefully, as they have an exceptionally delicate skeletal structure and can be injured very easily if improperly handled or dropped, especially susceptible to lumbar spinal luxation, resulting in paralysis. **Most rabbits get very uneasy when they are picked up and may struggle and hit you with its claws. Their hind legs are long and strong and their claws are curved and sharp like an eagle's.**

Young rabbits can be picked up by the skin of their neck, like a kitten, then placed on your hand, held up against your chest, with the other hand then cupping it around the tail area. As they grow bigger and heavier they don't like being picked up that way. Remove the adult rabbit from its cage by grasping the skin over the shoulders with one hand, turning the rabbit slightly to one side, and slowly pulling it to the front and lifting it out of the cage. Always support the rabbit's hindquarters by placing your hand around the rump (Fig. 0-5). Caution: If their feet dangle they kick around and can scratch. Rabbits must never by lifted by the ears.

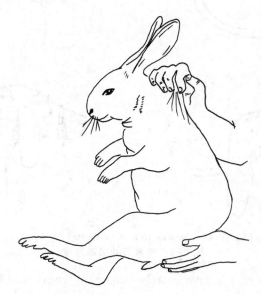

Fig. 0-5　The way to carry a rabbit
图 0-5　抓捕兔的姿势

(3) Measuring its body weight

(4) Securing the animal on an operative table

Things you'll need for the securing an animal are an operative table and four cotton threads for tying the legs. Operative table is a flat board or trough with cleats on the four corners for securing restraint cords, An assistant may be very helpful, and chemical restraint with ketamine is recommended to reduce struggling. The rabbit or dog is stretched out on its back with its hocks tied to the corner cleats. The abdomen is clipped and the skin cleaned with detergent.

4. Skin sutures are often unnecessary. They may cause the animal to chew or scratch at the incision site. **Alternatives include use of subcutaneous/intradermal closure techniques**

or tissue adhesive.

By the end of the operation, the wound would be left exposed to the air without dressings. The unconscious animal(s) should be kept away from their compatible animals and in clean, warm and dry board during the anesthetic-recovery phase.

Important Note:

Be sure to gently check the sutures for a day or two after surgery to be sure the rabbit isn't chewing them, and to check for unusual redness, swelling or signs of infection.

Offer your rabbit a bowl of water, even if a water bottle is usually used. A rabbit needs to drink after surgery, but often won't do so if he has to "work" for his/her water. He will recover more quickly if he's well hydrated.

Monitor the output of fecal pellets closely. If fecal output slows or stops after surgery, your rabbit may be suffering from GI stasis (ileus) due to the stress of the surgery.

E. ANESTHESIA

Good anesthesia practice consists of preventing awareness of pain in a controllable and reversible fashion with a minimum of risk during surgical procedure. Pentobarbital, thiopental, ketamine and ether have become the agents of choice for anesthesia in dog and rabbit, because they are effective, easily administered and inexpensive. Even though isoflurane gas is more expensive than injectable anesthetics and ether anesthetic, it is worth the extra cost to ensure a safer surgery and faster recovery.

1. Sodium pentobarbital: One of the commonly used intravenous agents is pentobarbital, which is yellow powder and should be dissolved in normal saline to the concentration of 2 per cent before use. Pentobarbital can be administered by two routes:

(1) Intravenous anesthesia: Rabbits are usually anesthetized with an intravenous dose of sodium pentobarbitone (30~60 mg/kg) via the marginal ear vein. Within 2~4 minutes the animal will lose consciousness, although it may experience a brief period of excitement. Anesthesia from pentobarbital can last from 1 to 2 hours, depending on the dose given. Additional amounts about one fifth to one fourth of initial dose can be given as necessary to maintain anesthesia, being careful not to overdose. The animal's physiological status should be monitored at regular intervals throughout the anesthesia, and antidote (cocculin) is prepared in case any complications occurred. One of the most useful indicators for measuring depth of anesthesia is heart rate (HR). When the jaw muscle tone is relaxed, the animal should be intubated. Please be aware that intubation of rabbits is a delicate procedure requiring a great deal of practice and expertise.

(2) Intraperitoneal anesthesia: Rabbits or dogs can be anesthetized with intraperitoneal injection of sodium pentobarbital at dosage of 40 mg/kg body weight. The onset of anesthesia state in intraperitoneal route is slower than intravenous administration.

The animal is usually restrained in dorsal recumbency. The operative board securing the animal is inclined slightly in a head down position. This position allows the intestines to fall toward the diaphragm and away from the injection site. Injections are made in the lateral aspect of the lower abdominal quadrants. However, it is best to try to avoid the left side in rabbits because of the presence of the cecum. After the needle is inserted, draw back. If anything is aspirated, you have likely hit the viscera: a distended urinary bladder (clear to yellowish fluid), the bowel (greenish-brown material), or the liver (blood). If the needle is placed correctly the drug may be injected. Drug administered into the viscera may result in no effect or in a complication.

2. Sodium thiopental: Thiopental is an ultrashort-acting sedative, which is dissolved in normal saline at 2.5 per cent concentration. Care must be taken to avoid perivascular or subcutaneous injection, which may cause significant tissue necrosis and skin sloughing, as thiopental is highly alkaline (pKa 10.5). Its dosage is determined by body weight but obese animals may require higher doses of thiopental to induce anesthesia. Anesthesia induced by this drug is associated with respiratory depression or apnea if the dose given is large. The administration routes are:

(1) Intravenous anesthesia: Rabbits or dogs are usually anesthetized with an intravenous dose of thiopental (15~20 mg/kg). It causes onset of unconsciousness in 1~2 minutes. Additional dosage about one fourth to one third of initial dose can be supplemented as needed, being careful not to overdose as described above under "sodium pentobarbital".

(2) Intraperitoneal anesthesia: Rabbits or dogs can be anesthetized with intraperitoneal injection of thiopental at dosage of 25 mg/kg body weight. The onset of anesthesia state in intraperitoneal route is slower than intravenous administration. If sedation is insufficient intraoperatively, 1/2 of the original dose is given intraperitonealy with the fascia grasped and lifted on either side of the incision with Allis.

(3) Intramuscular anesthesia: Dogs can be anesthetized with intramuscular dose of 25 mg/kg body weight thiopental applied by hand injection into the rear leg muscles. The onset of anesthesia state in this route is approximately in 5 to 7 minutes. If sedation is insufficient, 1/3 to 1/2 of the original dose is given in the same route.

3. Ketamine: Ketamine, known as a dissociative anesthetic, provides poor analgesic activity, especially for visceral pain. This drug is easy to use and have a wide margin of safety for most laboratory species. The animal's eyes will usually remain open and the corneas should be protected with a layer of ophthalmic petrolatum or other suitable ointment.

(1) Intravenous anesthesia: After the administration of 1 percent solution at 2 to 3 mg per kilogram intravenously, the animal rapidly becomes lack of response to stimuli and the anesthesia can last for 10~15 min. Additional dose (up to 10 mg per kilogram of total dose) can be given as necessary to maintain anaesthesia.

(2) Intramuscular anesthesia: After the administration of 2.5%~5% solution at 6~12 mg per kilogram intramuscularly, the animal becomes lack of response to stimuli and the anesthesia can last for 30 min. Additional dose up to 30 mg per kilogram of total dose

can be given as necessary to maintain anaesthesia. Rats can be anesthetized with ketamine (150 mg/kg, I. M.). Intramuscular and intraperitoneal injections of the dissociative anesthetics can be painful, as the drug is very acidic.

4. Ketamine-based combined anesthesia

In general, by mixing anesthetic and analgesic or sedative drugs, the dose required for each individual drug is reduced. Do not mix drugs in the syringe until you have determined that they are compatible when mixed. If in doubt, administer separately.

(1) Ketamine-Xylazine: This combination is effective, easily administered and inexpensive. For immobilization and painful procedures of pigs or dogs, the doses of 10 ∼ 15 mg/kg ketamine and 1∼3 mg/kg xylazine are generally required injecting intramuscularly by hand, as physically restraining these animals is both difficult and dangerous and may cause undue physiological stress to the animals. Because it is more difficult to estimate weights of these animals, we recommend erring toward heavier weight estimates when immobilizing these animals.

Rabbits can be anesthetized intramuscularly with ketamine (35 mg/kg) and xylazine (5 mg/kg) with or without acepromazine (0. 75 mg/kg).

(2) Ketamine-Medetomidine: Rabbits can be immobilized using a mixture of ketamine and medetomidine either subcutaneously or intramuscularly. The target dose was 5∼7 mg of Ketamine per kilogram of body weight combined with 0. 08 mg/kg of medetomidine.

5. Urethane (ethyl carbamate): After the administration of 20 percent solution at 5 ml per kilogram intravenously, the animal rapidly becomes lack of response to stimuli and the anesthesia can last for 50∼60 min, or even longer.

概　述

　　外科手术是治疗疾病的一种方法,尽管它的种类繁多,范围、大小和复杂程度有很大差别,但其基本操作相同。切开、显露、分离、止血、结扎、缝合既是手术的基本操作,也是做好手术的条件之一,其重要性就不言而喻了。《外科基本操作》这一课程,旨在通过模拟器具和动物手术实习,使学生建立无菌观念,并初步掌握手术的基本技术操作。

　　外科基本操作实验室是为学生学习外科基本操作提供必要的器械、设备和场所,为学生掌握好这门基本技术提供支持条件,为以后的临床学习打下基础。

　　学生进入实习室学习动物手术,应当同进入医院手术室做手术一样,不能认为是做动物手术而在思想上有所轻视。在整个实习中,必须严格遵守无菌操作规则,认真、细致地进行操作,爱护动物,防止麻醉意外、感染和动物死亡。

一、实习须知

　　1. 穿工作服,方可进入实习室。

　　2. 在隔离线处换拖鞋。

　　3. 在更衣室戴口罩和帽子,脱去自身的普通衣裤,换上手术衣和手术裤,然后才能进入手术室。帽子要求能完全遮住头发、头皮和鬓角(图 0-1)。口罩要盖住鼻孔,如果水汽雾了你的眼镜,可以在口罩的上缘、鼻两侧压一下,或在镜片上抹一层肥皂液,再擦净。然后,褪去内衣、裤,换穿手术室的洗手衣、裤。洗手衣应束在裤子内(图 0-2)。洗手衣、裤的材质应该是棉织品,不应该用化纤织品,以免产生静电,引燃麻醉气体。禁止将日常穿的衣裤穿入手术室的无菌区(限制区)或半无菌区(半限制区)。

　　4. 必须严肃认真,服从教师指导,禁止大声谈笑或喊叫。

　　5. 手术是一种团队工作,既要分工明确,又要相互合作,体现团队协作精神。

　　6. 手术要集中注意力,有高度责任心,尽管是动物操作,也不可草率从事。

　　7. 手术完毕后,将用过的器械洗净、消毒、擦干、上油、包好,放在规定处待灭菌。

　　8. 离开手术室前,手术人员应该脱下手套、帽、口罩和手术衣,分别放入指定的容器内。

　　9. 厉行节约,保持整洁,爱护公物。

　　10. 外科打结需要课后勤练,才能逐渐运用自如,因此,学生们起初几次的课后作业就是打结。外科技巧的学习需要时间,开始应力求方法正确,不要图快,通过反复练习,速度和效率自然会长进。进入动物手术实习后,由麻醉者记录麻醉情况,手术者写实习报告(包括手术记录、术后观察记录等),其方法见附录三。学生在完成本门课程的学习后,其成绩将根据下列技巧的熟练程度进行评分:打结、无菌术(洗手、戴手套和穿无菌手术衣)、心肺复苏以及医疗文件的书写。

二、手术实习时的人员分工

手术室的人员都有明确的分工,因此,在动物试验阶段,学生将以小组为单位进行操作。同学之间应该齐心协力,为手术的成功而努力。

1. 手术者(主刀)　根据实习要求负责做手术(切开、分离、止血、结扎、缝合),是手术组的主导人物。手术时通常站在病人或动物的右边(图 0-3)。

2. 第一助手　应先洗手,负责手术区皮肤的消毒和协助铺巾。手术时站在手术者对面,负责止血、擦(吸)血,协助完成手术。

3. 第二助手　根据手术的需要,可站在手术者或第一助手的左侧。负责拉钩(显露)、剪线等工作。

4. 手术护士　最先洗手,安排好手术器械,站在手术者的旁边(相当于病人大腿的位置),负责传递手术需要的一切器械、线、敷料、液体和药品;缝合时,将针穿好线后递给手术者;维持手术区的清洁;并在手术结束前与巡回护士共同核对器械、缝针和纱布的数目。

所有可能被遗留在创口内的物品都应该按规定由两人清点,并在记录单上写下纱球、针、各种器械等的数目,该过程简称为点数。要求在手术开始前点出基数,在体腔缝合前和皮肤缝合前复点。

5. 麻醉师　负责麻醉和观察麻醉情况,调整生命体征,兼管输液。如发生变化应设法急救,并通知手术者。

6. 巡回护士　负责准备和供应工作,随时供应需要的物品。把污物桶放在无菌区附近供丢弃污物用。参与清点、记录和核对手术器械、缝针和纱布等。协助手术人员穿好手术衣。

三、实验动物的准备

在我们学校,一般用狗或兔作为外科基本操作实习的动物。

1. 有条件者,手术前一周将动物从饲养场转到实验场所的动物房内,以免动物因环境突然改变而感到不安或厌食,以致影响实验。同时也可和工作人员熟悉,进行手术前必要的治疗和准备。

2. 对于狗和猫来说,手术前夜,除给水外,不喂任何食物(禁食,不禁饮),以免手术时呕吐和误吸,同时便于腹部手术的显露和操作。但是,兔手术前不主张禁食,因为兔没有呕吐反射,此外,短时间的肠道空虚就会造成肝损害,好在兔胃肠道的排空时间很长。

3. 动物的捕捉和制动

(1) 狗的抓捕远比兔困难。一般用捕狗笼将狗挤在狭窄的空间里,也可用专用套狗器将狗控制,在其后腿肌内注射氯胺酮或乙酰普马嗪,待其不能动弹。然后,捆绑鼻口部和四肢。狗鼻口的捆绑应松紧适度,既不会松脱被狗咬伤,也不造成狗的不适。市场上有各种大小的口套出售,但我们一般按下法捆绑狗的鼻口(图 0-4):

取一段 1 m 长、1~1.5 cm 宽的布带绳,用两手分别提着该绳的两端,打一个松的单结,制成一个绳圈。将绳圈套过狗的下颌,在上颌上把结打紧;然后,转向下颌再打一个结;接着,将绳索引至两侧耳后在颈项部打第三个结,在第三个结上再打一个蝴蝶结固定。**所有**

的结都必须打牢,但也不要因过紧而勒伤狗的皮肤,造成狗的不适或挣扎。

卸去绳套的方法是在颈项部解开蝴蝶结,再解开下颌下的一个结。此时,两手要远离狗嘴,轻轻地牵动绳索松动上颌上的结,慢慢地脱下口套,切勿强行拉扯。

若术中发现狗有呼吸困难或呕吐,应该立即松开狗的口套。

(2)兔的骨骼结构很脆弱,不恰当地抓起或扔下很容易造成损伤,尤其腰椎容易发生脱位,导致截瘫,因此,兔的抓捕要轻柔。大多数兔子会变得不安,可能会挣扎并用爪子抓人。此外,**兔的后爪极为尖利,随意抓取时很容易遭致抓伤。**

幼兔体重小,可以用一只手抓住颈部的皮肤拎起,另一只手托住兔臀部抱起。体重增加或成年兔则不能如此拎起,可以先用一只手抓住颈部的皮肤,但兔腿不离地,然后用另一只手托住兔臀部或抓住两后腿将兔从笼子里取出来,抱起(图0-5)。注意:不要让兔的腿悬空,以免挣扎时受伤。绝对不能抓住兔的两耳将兔拎起。

(3)称体重。

(4)把动物固定于手术台上:固定动物的手术台面最好有个浅凹槽,手术台的四个角各有一个固定拴,供系绳索用。另外,需准备四根棉绳,用于束缚动物的四肢。固定动物最好请一位同学协助,并在氯胺酮麻醉下进行,减少动物的痛苦和惊慌。将动物仰躺在手术台上,用绳索固定四肢踝部,然后开始在腹部剪毛、清洗。

4. 动物手术后一般不主张缝合皮肤,因为动物会咬或抓切口。可以用皮内缝合法或用组织胶粘合。

手术完毕,不需包扎伤口,可任其暴露。麻醉未醒前,最好将动物单独安放在清洁、温暖和干燥处。

重要提示:

术后最初两天,要检查缝线是否已被咬掉,伤口有无红肿等感染征象。

在兔的身边放一碗水,因为吸吮瓶装水需要体力。手术后的兔需要饮水,饮水有益于康复。

密切观察兔的粪粒,若兔在手术后排粪延迟或不排便,提示手术造成了兔的肠麻痹。

四、动物的麻醉

一个好的麻醉不但能够止痛,具有可控性和可逆性,而且风险小,从而保证手术顺利进行。用狗或兔做实验动物时,多采用戊巴比妥钠、硫喷妥钠、氯胺酮或乙醚作麻醉剂,比较经济和安全,便于管理。有些动物手术可以选用异氟烷吸入麻醉,它比注射麻醉剂及乙醚更安全,恢复更快,然而价格高昂。

1. 戊巴比妥钠麻醉 先将戊巴比妥钠结晶溶于灭菌生理盐水中,配制成2%的溶液备用。根据给药途径,可分为:

(1)静脉麻醉:在兔耳廓背面耳缘选定一条静脉,消毒皮肤后,按30~60 mg/kg的剂量,从静脉内缓慢注入戊巴比妥钠溶液。一般在注射后2~4分钟即出现麻醉状态,有时会有短时间躁动,通常可以维持麻醉1~2小时。如在手术过程中发现麻醉不够深,可以再注射原剂量的1/5~1/4,要注意避免麻醉剂过量。麻醉剂过量发生呼吸和循环抑制时,可用人工呼吸和静脉注射印防己毒素3 mg来急救。麻醉过程中要定时监测生命体征,尤其是心率。下颌松弛时应及时做气管插管。注意:兔的气管插管需要相当的技巧,动作要轻柔。

（2）腹腔内麻醉：按 40 mg/kg，将戊巴比妥钠溶液注入腹腔内，通过腹膜的吸收而达到麻醉，但起效较为缓慢。

腹腔内麻醉需要行腹腔穿刺，动物一般先仰卧固定于手术台上，将手术台调至头低位，使腹腔内脏上移。然后，在腹部脐下一侧进行穿刺。兔要避免从左下腹进针，以免刺入巨大的盲肠。进针后，要回抽，观察有无液体抽出，防止误入膨胀的膀胱（黄色液）、肠道（绿色液）或肝脏（血性液）。待明确针的位置正确进入腹腔后才开始注入麻醉剂。麻醉剂误入内脏可造成麻醉失效，或引起并发症。

2. 硫喷妥钠麻醉　硫喷妥钠是一种超短效麻醉剂，一般将硫喷妥钠结晶溶于灭菌生理盐水中配制成 2.5% 的溶液备用。硫喷妥钠碱性大，因此切勿注入血管外或皮下，以免发生皮肤和组织坏死。硫喷妥钠麻醉的剂量，个体差异大，术中易发生呼吸抑制，不易掌握，不如戊巴比妥钠安全。根据给药途径，可分为：

（1）静脉麻醉：按 15～20 mg/kg 的剂量，从静脉内缓慢注入硫喷妥钠溶液。通常 1～2 分钟即出现麻醉作用，如麻醉不深，则补加原剂量的 1/4～1/3，或以 0.1% 的浓度静脉滴注加深麻醉。麻醉切忌过量。手术中如发生呼吸抑制，抢救方法同戊巴比妥钠。

（2）腹腔内注射：将 25 mg/kg 的硫喷妥钠注入腹腔内，出现麻醉作用比静脉注入慢。术中麻醉变浅，动物出现躁动时，可将切口两缘用 Allis 钳或拉钩提起，于腹内滴入原剂量的 1/2，术者用手轻揉腹部片刻，促使药液扩散、吸收。

（3）肌内注射：以 25 mg/kg 的硫喷妥钠注入臀部肌肉内，5～7 分钟即出现麻醉作用。如麻醉不深，可追加原剂量的 1/3～1/2。

3. 氯胺酮麻醉　盐酸氯胺酮是一种分离麻醉剂，对内脏疼痛的止痛作用不理想。本药使用方便，对大多数动物都安全，为其优点。麻醉中，动物通常是睁眼的，因此，要用凡士林或其他软膏涂抹保护角膜。

（1）静脉麻醉：用 1% 溶液，按 2～3 mg/kg 静注，可维持麻醉 10～15 分钟，之后根据需要追加，总量可达 10 mg/kg。

（2）肌内注射：用 2.5%～5% 溶液，按 6～12 mg/kg 肌注，可维持麻醉 30 分钟，以后根据需要追加，总量可达 30 mg/kg。大鼠肌内麻醉时剂量可达 150 mg/kg。氯胺酮的酸度强，肌内注射或腹腔注射都会引起疼痛。

4. 含氯胺酮的静脉复合麻醉

麻醉剂与止痛剂或镇静剂合用，可以减少这些药的用量。但是，在你确定这些药允许配伍之前，千万不要把它们抽在一个注射器内混合，要分开用。

（1）氯胺酮—甲苯噻嗪方案：该方案具有效果好、使用方便、价格便宜等优点。氯胺酮 10～15 mg/kg 和甲苯噻嗪 1～3 mg/kg，肌内注射，主要用于狗、猪等大动物的捕捉困难时或有危险性时。由于动物的体重估计往往难以正确，我们主张将动物的体重高估，以达到制动的目的。

兔可以用氯胺酮 35 mg/kg 加甲苯噻嗪各 5 mg/kg，肌内注射麻醉，加或不加乙酰普马嗪 0.75 mg/kg。

（2）氯胺酮—美托咪定方案：用 5～7 mg/kg 加美托咪定 0.08 mg/kg，肌内注射或皮下注射，主要用于兔的麻醉。

5. 乌拉坦（氨基甲酸乙酯）　用 20% 溶液，按 5 ml/kg 静注，可维持麻醉 50～60 分钟，甚至更长时间。

Session 1　Surgical aseptic techniques &
Basic surgical knot making

【Goals & requirements】

1. Clearly distinguishing among hygiene, sterile, nonsterile, and aseptic.

2. Understand the rationale for practicing aseptic technique and practice the rules of aseptic technique, including the surgical hand scrub, donning gown and gloves, skin preparation and draping.

3. Correctly master surgical knot tying.

【Progress schedule】

1. Students are divided into two groups; the students assigned to Block A learns aseptic technique and students in Block B knot tying. After 2 hours, the two groups exchange their tasks each other.

2. Educator will demonstrate the techniques first, and then students will be asked to follow step by step.

【Topics of this session】

A. Surgical aseptic techniques

（A）preoperative preparation of sterile team members

1. Surgical Attire

（1）Change into OR (operating room) shoes at the barrier; apply shoe covers, if necessary.

（2）Apply OR hair cover and mask, as needed.

（3）Don scrub suit.

（4）Keep nails short and trim the nails, if necessary.

2. Surgical Scrub

The most common cause of surgical site infection is the normal bacteria found on the skin of the patient and surgical team members, particularly Staphylococcus aureus. Skin is colonized by both superficial (transient) bacteria, which are easily removed by soap and water, and deep (permanent or resident) bacteria (Fig. 1-1) that live in deeper skin structures such as sweat and sebaceous glands, and hair follicles, which cannot be destroyed by surgical skin antiseptics. The surgical scrub does not sterilize the skin and it is to reduce the number of transient microorganisms to an absolute minimum. Bacteria proliferate quickly in the moist environment between the skin and glove and surgeon's hand will show just as high a bacterial count at the end of an operation as they did before scrubbing began. It becomes clear, therefore, that surgical scrub alone is not enough.

(1) Handwashing with soap

① Perform routine washing of hands and arms using plain soap. **The effectiveness of soap depends on friction to remove organic and inorganic matter from skin.** Rinse hands and arms thoroughly under running water.

② Obtain a sterile brush and soaked it in sterile liquid soap. Scrub hands extending to 10 centimeters above the elbow. Avoid harsh friction with the brush because it may scratch skin. Repeated skin irritation encourages colonization of both resident and transient bacteria on the hands and arms. **Pay attention to scrubbing the nails, the interdigital spaces, and the wrists.**

When performing the surgical scrub, begin with all of the nails and cuticles by placing the fingertips together and proceed to the radial, back and ulnar sides of the thumb, the same three sides of rest fingers, palm, back of hand, wrists and arms, without returning to a previously scrubbed area (Fig. 1-2).

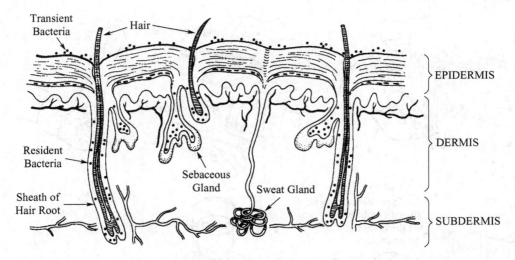

Fig. 1-1 Lovell's concept of the transient bacteria and resident bacteria
图 1-1 Lovell 皮肤暂驻菌和常驻菌的概念

③ Rinse from fingertips to the elbows under running water. Discard the brush, have a fresh one and begin the second time of scrubbing. It is recommended that a scrub should be thrice and 3 minutes each time for soap handwashing. Keep hands higher than elbows at all times by holding the elbows bent so that water runs from the tips of the fingers toward the elbows (Fig. 1-2-4). The times and length of the scrub should be the same for both the initial surgical scrub and all scrubs that follow during the day. Try to remove residual suds from back aspect of your elbows.

If using the counted method, scrub the nails and hand with 20 strokes (one stroke is the combined back and forth motion), then the other. Proceed to the four surfaces of one arm (10 strokes on each surface) and then the other.

Do not allow the scrubbed hand or arm to contact any part of the sink, faucet, or scrub suit. Avoid splashing water on the scrub suit.

Before operation, the hands and forearms should be cleansed and scrubbed thoroughly with an antimicrobial soap for at least 5 minutes for the first case or after any dirty case and for 3 minutes for subsequent cases, and then with a modern antiseptic solution.

④ Drying hands and arms with a towel (Fig. 1-2-5). Pick up a folded sterile towel with the fingers of both hands. Allow the towel to unfold so that the long edge hangs down between your two hands. Use one end of the towel to dry one hand and arm, working from hand to wrist to elbow without moving back over a previously dried area, and then use the other end for the other hand and arm. If you only have small size towel, pick up one for one hand and arm, and then second for the other. Dry hands by blotting with a towel and drying the arm using the blotting rotating motion. Try not to bring the towel beyond the area of scrub. Do not allow the towel to contact the scrub suit. The towel may be discarded in the linen hamper.

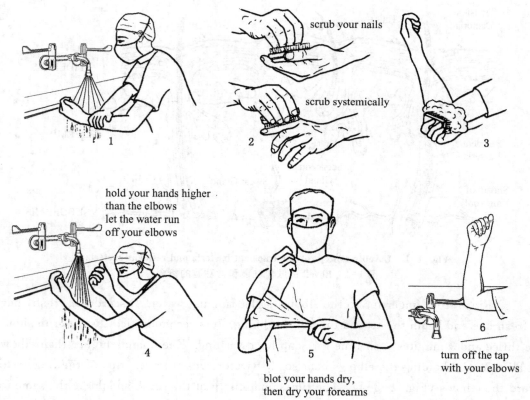

Fig. 1-2　Surgical scrub and drying
图 1-2　外科洗手和揩手法

⑤ Alcohol or Benzalkonium Bromide dip: Alcohol at 75 per cent concentration and Benzalkonium Bromide at 0.1 per cent concentration are very effective skin antiseptics. Soak your hands extending to 6 centimeters above the elbow for 5 minutes in a basin containing an antiseptic, bacterial counts are rapidly and dramatically reduced; and the application of friction with a gauze square gives even better results. Note and avoid your hands or forearm touching the edge of the bucket which is unsterile when you withdraw your hands from the bucket.

⑥ Hold your hands higher than your elbows immediately when you withdraw them from the basin and allow the excess antiseptic solution to drop into the basin.

(2) Handwashing with disinfectant: Wet your hands thoroughly under running water and apply a little plain soap and work up a good lather. Rub your hands and forearms to 10 cm above your elbows for one complete minute. Rinsed with running water.

Scrub hands and arms using brush with a disinfectant such as povidone iodine or chlorhexidine for 3 minutes or with alcohol-based preparation for at least 60 sec. Rub the hands together vigorously including the backs of the hands, interdigital spaces, and wrists. To ensure that the spaces between the fingers are adequately washed. Rinse all disinfectant from hands and forearms.

Hold your hands higher than your elbows and allow the excess water to drop into the sink. Proceed directly to the operating room. Enter by pushing the door open with your back or hip. Proceed to drying, gowning, and gloving.

3. Gowning and gloving

(1) Gowning. When gowning, consider the gown as having two surfaces: an inside surface that will contact the nonsterile scrub suit and bare skin of hands and arms, and an outside surface that will be considered sterile. It has been folded so that the inside faces out and the outside faces inward, and your bare scrubbed hand is allowed to pick it up.

Grasp the gown and bring it away from the table and nonsterile facilities. Identify collar and orient gown. Holding the inside of the gown near the shoulders, high enough to be well above the floor, allow it to unfold gently. Identify the arm openings and place hands inside the sleeves while keeping your arms extended. Then flex your elbows to hold gown in place. Wait for the circulating nurse to help you. She will grasp the inner sides of the gown at each shoulder and pull them over your shoulders, and secure the neck and inside fasteners. At last, cross your arms and hand the waist tab to the circulator who will secure for you (Fig. 1-3). Notice: slightly bent your body forward and suspend the waist ties before you pick them up in order to avoid touching the gown.

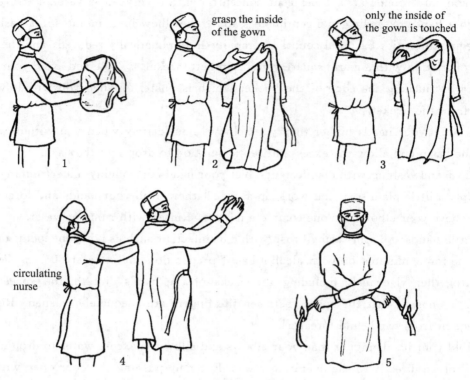

grasp the inside of the gown

only the inside of the gown is touched

circulating nurse

Fig. 1-3 Gowning
图 1-3 穿无菌手术衣法

(2) Open gloving technique: The open gloving technique is used during sterile procedures that do not require donning a sterile gown, such as urinary catheterization and patient skin preparation. The hands are not usually scrubbed before open gloving, although they always should be washed.

When gloving, think of the glove as having two surfaces: the inside and the outside. Before the gloves are touched, the both sides are sterile. As soon as gloving is initiated, however, the inside surface is considered nonsterile. **Be careful to touch only the inner surface of the gloves with ungloved hand.** It has been folded so that each glove has a cuff that exposes the inside surface of the glove, and your bare scrubbed hand is allowed to touch the exposed side of the cuff.

Open the glove wrapper (sterilized, which has been delivered by circulator) with bare hands and expose the gloves. Orient the palms of the glove upward, thumbs outward. Pick up a glove by its cuffed edge with one hand, and pull it on to your opposite hand without touching the glove exterior. Leave its cuff for the moment until you glove the other hand.

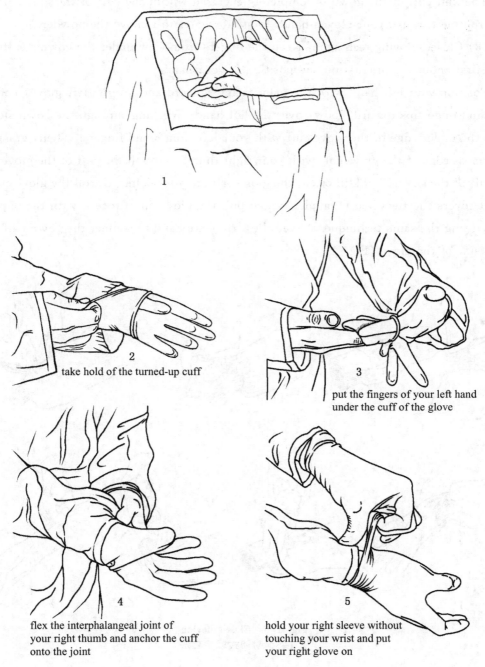

1

2
take hold of the turned-up cuff

3
put the fingers of your left hand
under the cuff of the glove

4
flex the interphalangeal joint of
your right thumb and anchor the cuff
onto the joint

5
hold your right sleeve without
touching your wrist and put
your right glove on

Fig. 1-4　Open gloving
图 1-4　开放式戴手套法

Put the fingers of your already gloved hand under the inverted cuff of the other glove,
and pull it onto the bare hand. Do not allow the gloved hand to touch any bare skin and

keep the gloved thumb well out of the way(Fig. 1-4).

The knit cuff of the gown is completely enclosed within the cuff of the glove. It is a good routine to wash your gloved hands in sterile water to remove the powder.

(3) Closed gloving technique: Keep the fingers from view under the gown's cuffs and think first about the orientation and position of your hand.

Position your left hand with the palm facing upward and lay the left glove, palm to palm and fingertips toward elbow, over the left hand. Working through the gown sleeve, grasp the under edge of the glove cuff with your left thumb and fingers. Then, grasp the uppermost edge of the glove cuff with your right thumb and pull the cuff of the glove over the cuff of the gown, but still orient the glove palm to your palm. Unroll the glove cuff so that it covers the sleeve cuff completely and pull the glove on. Proceed with the opposite hand, using the same technique. Never allow the bare hand to contact the gown cuff edge or outside of the glove (Fig. 1-5).

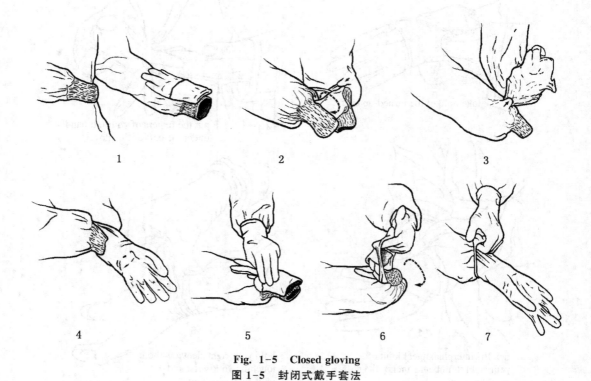

Fig. 1-5　Closed gloving
图 1-5　封闭式戴手套法

(4) Gloving another: The first person to glove up (usually the scrub nurse) now helps the next person (usually the surgeon) who has gowned on with their gloves (Fig. 1-6).

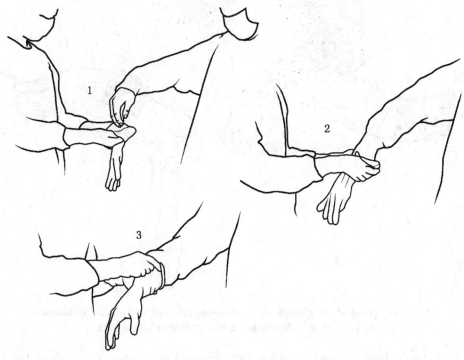

Fig. 1-6   Gloving another

1. Pick up the right glove and place the palm away from you. Slide the fingers under the glove cuff and spread them so that a wide opening is created. Keep thumbs under the cuff. 2. The surgeon thrusts his or her hand into the glove. Do not release the glove yet. 3. Gently release the cuff (do not let the cuff snap sharply) while unrolling it over the wrist. Proceed with the left glove, using the same technique.

图 1-6   为他人戴手套

1. 助手先拿右手套,手套的掌面朝外,两手的手指伸入手套反折部内拉撑手套使手套口张开。拇指也要插入手套反折部内。2. 外科医生将手插入手套。助手不要松开手套。3. 慢慢将手套的反折部上翻套于腕部,用力过大会撕破手套。然后,按相同的方法为他/她戴左侧手套。

(5) Glove removal for replacement during a procedure:

① If you tear or contaminate a glove during an operation, remove it. Grasp its cuff from the outside with your opposite hand, and pull it down over your palm by touching the outer side of the cuff only. Then, invert the other glove in the same way and remove it (Fig. 1-7). At last, remove the remaining glove by sliding the ungloved hand between the skin of palm and the glove, so it is removed to contain both gloves.

② Gown and glove removal for replacement during a procedure: If contamination occurs during a procedure, both gown and gloves may be discarded and new gown and gloves must be added as follows. Remain with your back to the circulator so that the grown can be unfastened. Face the circulator and maintain an appropriate distance from her while she removes the gown for you. Then, extend both arms with the palms upward to allow the circulator to grasp the glove exteriors and remove them. Rescrub, if necessary, and don new gown and gloves.

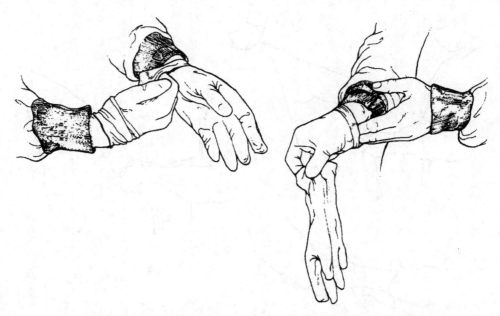

Fig. 1-7　Take off surgical gloves by glove-to-glove and skin-to-skin technique
图 1-7　手套—手套接触、皮肤—皮肤接触的脱手套法

③ Gown and glove removal at end of procedure: The circulator unfastens the back of the gown and you may remove the gown inside out by grasping the gown near shoulders. Then, the gloves are removed using glove-to-glove, then skin-to-skin technique.

（B） Preparation of the patient

1. Skin prep of surgical field

（1） It is the circulator's job to pick the animal up from cages or kennel and clip hair short after anesthesia. There is usually no need to shave a patient unless the hair at or around the incision site will interfere with the operation. If hair is removed, remove immediately before the operation, preferably with electric clippers. Depilatory cream may be preferred, particularly if large areas need to be shaved.

（2） It is the first assistant's job to perform surgical skin preparation following his or her scrubbing up, usually before his or her gowning and gloving.

（3） Traditionally, skin preparation starts with a single application of alcoholic iodine at 3 percent, and left to it dry and then three with alcohol at 75 percent are used to remove iodine. Be sure to prepare a wide enough area of skin, at least 20 cm from incision.

Alcohol destroys microorganisms through desiccation of the cell proteins. For this reason, alcohol and alcohol-based antiseptics, especially alcoholic iodine, should not be used on the vagina, cervix, rectum or other mucous membranes, infants skin, or perineum skin because they easily irritate these tissues. As a result, 0.5 percent of ionosphere and chlorhexidine are popular recently. Effective cleansing requires both mechanical and chemical action, **so enough friction must be applied to cleanse the skin.** The process is repeated thrice for at least 5 minutes.

(4) Scrubbing should start at the center of the surgical site and move to the outside in a linear (Fig. 1-8) or circular manner (Fig. 1-9). A soiled sponge must never be brought back over a scrubbed area.

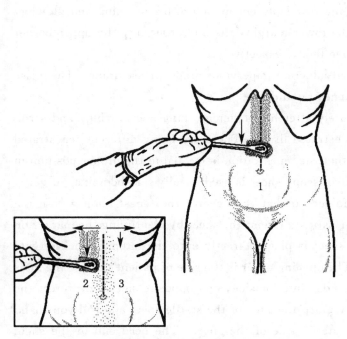

Fig. 1-8   Abdominal preparation (linear manner)
图 1-8   腹部皮肤的消毒(纵向)

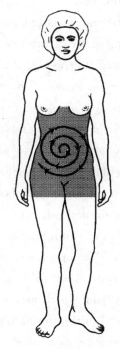

Fig. 1-9   Abdominal preparation
(circular manner)
图 1-9   腹部皮肤的消毒
(等进螺线方向)

When prepping the area of infection or anus, cover the area with a sponge soaked in the antiseptic solution first and prep the area last. A sponge is wiped in a circular motion too, but from periphery toward center. Each sponge should be discarded after going over the contaminated site.

2. Squaring off the incision and draping

After skin prep, the patient is covered with sterile surgical towels and procedure drape (sheet) that expose only the surgical site and create the center of the sterile field.

(1) It is the first assistant's job to frame the incision site and drape patient, usually after his or her gowning and gloving. The scrub nurse is responsible for surgical towel presentation. Towels are folded over at the top edge about one fourth of the width and one is presented to the surgeon at a time.

(2) Towels are placed 2~3 cm from incision with the folded edge facing the incision site and without contaminating the gloved hands. The first towel is placed on the side of

patient nearest the individual applying the drape, the second and the third inferiorly and superiorly, and the forth opposite the first towel. Clip the towels at their intersections with four towel clips. The principles of draping are that after the surgical towels have been placed, they can be moved from centre toward periphery, but can not be moved from periphery inward.

If the first assistant performs the towel placement before his gowning and gloving, the placing order of the towels is the lower margin, the lateral aspect, the upper border and the medial aspect of the operative field, respectively.

Cover the incision site with a self-adherent impervious drape (incise drape). The incise drape may also be placed over the fenestrated drape.

(3) It is the first assistant (surely after his or her gowning and gloving) and scrub nurse's cooperative job to place fenestrated drape. There are many different fenestrated drapes available, each designed so that the fenestration is located in the proper position in relation to the rest of the body. Laparoscopy sheet is used usually for abdominal surgery. Procedure drapes (sheets) are fanfolded so that they center the fenestration within the folds and can be unfolded easily over patient. Orient the sheet by identifying the marker on the sheet. The fenestration of the sheet is placed directly onto the intended incision site and then opened out fold by fold. The opening order is the side of patient nearest the individual applying the drape, superior side, inferior side, and opposite side. To protect the gloved hand during unfolding sheet, grasp the edge of the sterile sheet and roll your hand inward keeping your hands on the sterile side of the sheet. The head end of the sheet should cover anesthesia screen (headscreen), and the bilateral sides and the foot end of the sheet should hang below the table edge 31~40 cm.

(4) In order to avoid contamination, all people, except for the first assistant and the scrub, should keep away during the draping procedure. The first assistant and the scrub should remain a safe distance from the operating table to avoid contamination of your gown until the drapes have been applied. Drapes are not relocated after initial placement and misplaced drapes may be coved with another drape.

(C) Opening a small wrapped sterile package

Check the integrity of the packaging material. Unfold the outer packaging material with bare hand and orient the pack correctly on table. Unfold the inner packaging material with sterile ring forceps. Pull the top flap away from you. The side flaps are opened next in the appropriate directions, followed by the near flap toward you.

(D) The principle of asepsis during surgery

Creating and maintaining a sterile field is vital during surgery. Only sterile objects and personnel may be allowed within the sterile field. Every operating team member in the OR, sterile personnel or non sterile personnel, must rigorously abide by following principles.

1. The sterile field is kept in constant view. Verbally warn the scrub if a break in aseptic technique is identified or in question. "If in doubt, consider it contaminated." There should no reluctance on the part of any member of the surgical team to admit to a break in sterile technique. The member who hesitates or cannot carry through with this duty has no place in the OR. There can be no compromise of sterile technique in the OR.

2. When a sterile field is created around a procedure site, the sterile "zone" is considered such as: the front of the gown from the waist or table level to the mid-chest line, the gloves, the sleeves from 5 cm above the elbow to the cuff, table level and Mayo stand. Elbows are kept close to the sides to avoid touching nonsterile person, and hands are never placed in the axillary region (Fig. 1-10).

The nonsterile "zone" is considered such as: the back and shoulders of a wraparound-style gown, edges of a wrapper around a 5 cm perimeter, and drape below the table edge, be-

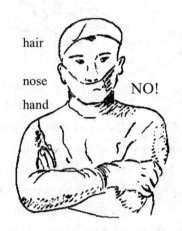

Fig. 1-10   Unacceptable manners during surgery
图 1-10   手术中不允许的举止

yond anesthesia screen and out of Mayo stand. Any item that extends beyond or below the table edge is considered nonsterile. If sterile person must stand on a platform, the platform should be positioned before the person approaches the sterile field, as moving from a lower position to a higher position within the field exposes contaminated areas of the gown to the field. A nonsterile individual or items must maintain a minimum of 30 cm of space from the sterile field or item.

Sterile instruments are not passed over nonsterile areas, such as the head or back of sterile person. Unsterile personnel are not allowed to reach across the sterile field.

3. Sterile personnel should stay close to and face to the sterile field throughout the procedure. Movement within the sterile field should be kept to a minimum. When stay position needs to be changed, the sterile persons pass each other back to back by rotation 360° (Fig. 1-11), or sterile person should turn her or his back to a nonsterile person or area when working past.

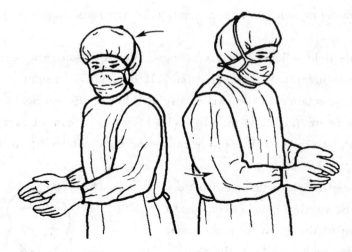

Fig. 1-11 Stay position change
图 1-11 无菌人员更换位置

4. The cloth drapes allow penetration by bacteria from a nonsterile to a sterile surface when wet because of capillary phenomena, the integrity of microbial barriers is destroyed and an impermeable towel with an adhesive edge should be placed over the site to maintain the sterile field. The gown should be replaced if the sleeves are wet from perspiration.

5. If the integrity of a glove is compromised (e. g. , punctured), it should be changed as promptly as safety permits. A study showed that as many as 18,960 staphylococci could pass through a single needle hole from the gloved finger in 20 minutes.

6. Instruments, such as scalpel blades, that come into contact with the skin of the patient should not be reused. During the course of the operation, if a hollow viscus is to be opened or other sources of contamination are to be exposed, protective gauze or plastic should be used to shield the adjacent normal tissues and separate setups should be used for the clean and dirty portions of the procedure. Personnel should not reuse the instruments used during the open hollow viscus or dirty portion of the procedure and should regown and reglove before returning to the use of sterile instruments from the clean setup.

7. Minimizing traffic flow and conversation in the operating room significantly reduces the risk of contamination of the surgical site. Face should turn to the nonsterile field to make cough or sneeze.

8. During the period of operation suspension, i. e. , waiting the frozen section report, the wound should be covered by sterile towel. Patient's arms should be well secured to avoid his hand touch the sterile field, if he is restlessness. Scrub the incision skin with a single application of alcohol before suture the skin.

9. Instruments or items can not be passed or taken each other between two sterile op-

eration tables.

10. Damaged tissue by crushing or drying heals slowly and is susceptible to infection. Gentle tissue handling, meticulous attention to effective hemostasis, and minimizing devitalized tissue and foreign bodies (i. e. , sutures, charred tissues) during surgery can reduce the risk of infection. When tying off vessels include only a minimum of surrounding tissues.

B. Basic surgical knot making

(A) Ligature is frequently used to achieve hemostasis in the operative field and to hold tissue together after suture, so correct method in knot tying is an important part of good surgical skills. Secure knots will prevent knot loose or slippage leading to bleeding or wound disruption the patient has to suffer or, even worse, threatening life.

The knot is the weakest portion of the suture. If the two ends of the suture are pulled in opposite directions with uniform rate and tension, so called "three points (the two ends of the suture and the knot) in one line", the knot may be tied more securely. Speed in tying knots may result in less than perfect placement of the strands.

Three-throw flat knots are appropriate for use in dermatologic surgery; however, the suture material may affect the number of throws needed for security. Extra throws do not increase the strength of a properly tied knot, but they do add to its bulk and, therefore, to any potential tissue reaction.

(B) Basic Knots for Surgery

1. Square knot: This is the easiest and most reliable for tying most suture materials including silk.

Caution: If the strands of a square knot are inadvertently incorrectly crossed (Fig. 1-12), a granny knot (Fig. 1-12) will result. Granny knots are not recommended because they have a tendency to slip when subjected to increased stress. Slip knot (Fig. 1-12) will form if one maintains traction on one end of the strand or the two ends of the suture are pulled with different tensions.

2. Extra half hitch on reef knot: With some synthetic materials, knot security requires the standard surgical technique of flat and square ties with additional throws (Fig. 1-12) if indicated by surgical circumstance and the experience of the surgeon.

3. Surgeon's knot or friction knot: Surgeon's knot is a double-wrap throw followed by a single throw which gives the knot additional friction to reduce slipping (Fig. 1-12).

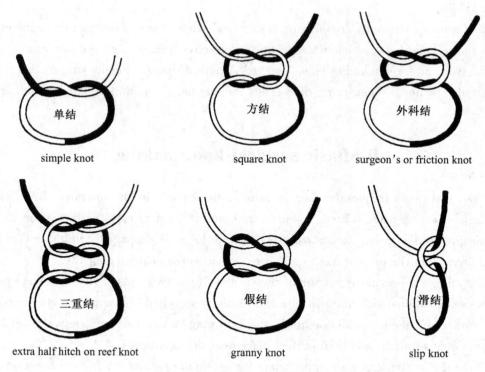

Fig. 1-12   Basic knots for surgery
图 1-12   外科常用结

(C) Techniques of knot tying

1. One-hand tie: The working strand is usually held in the right hand (Fig. 1-13). The left-handed person may choose to study the figures in a mirror. If you are not good in using your index finger when you make the second half hitch, a modified one-hand technique can be learned (Fig. 1-14).

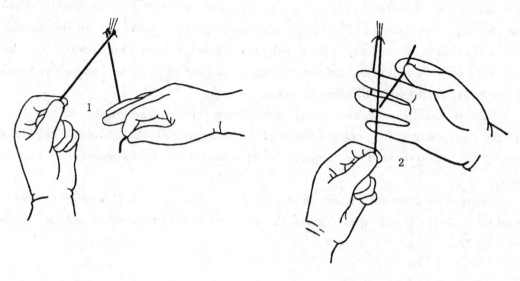

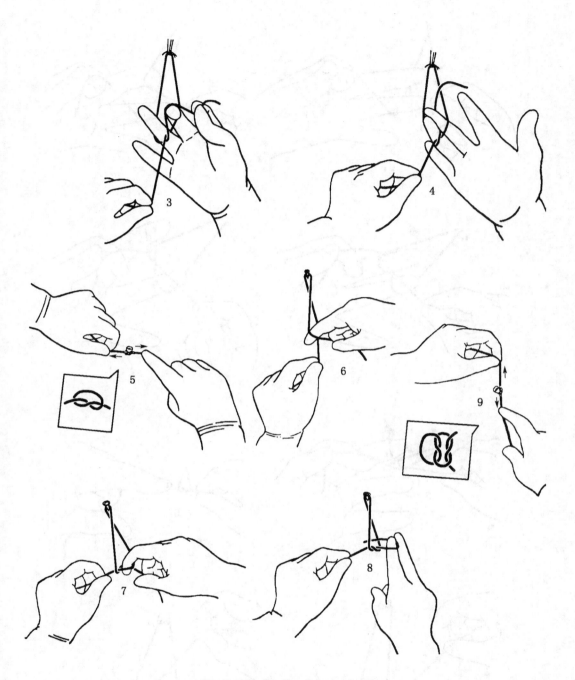

Fig. 1-13   One-hand square knot

In Step 1 one suture end is crossed over the other before beginning the tie. Hands are uncrossed at the end of the first loop tie (Step 5) but must be crossed after the second loop tie to produce a flat square knot (Step 9).

图 1-13   单手（右手）打结法

如 1 所示，两线头交叉开始打结，第一个结打紧时两手不交叉(5)；在第二个结打紧时两手要交叉(9)。

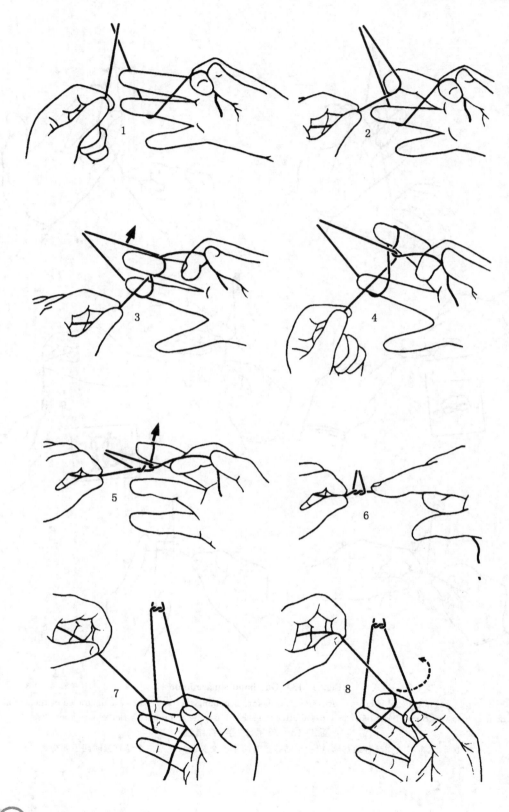

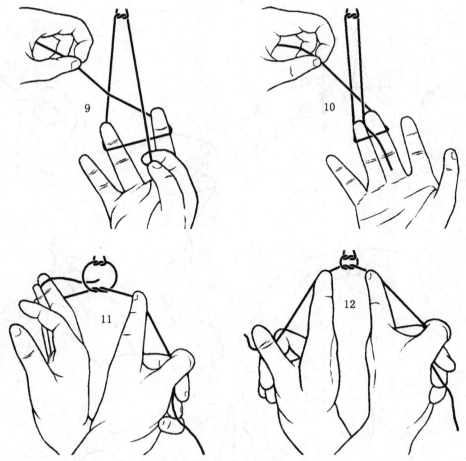

Fig. 1–14   A modified one-hand technique

In Step 1 one suture end is crossed over the other before beginning the tie. Hands are uncrossed at the end of the first loop tie (Step 6) but must be crossed after the second loop tie to produce a flat square knot (Step 12).

图 1–14   单手打结变式

如 1 所示,两线头交叉开始打结,第一个结打紧时两手不交叉(6);在第二个结打紧时两手要交叉(12)。

2. Two-hand tie (Fig. 1–15) is the easiest and most reliable for tying most suture materials. It may be used to tie surgical gut, virgin silk, surgical cotton, and surgical stainless steel.

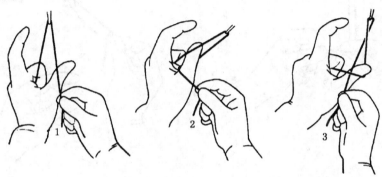

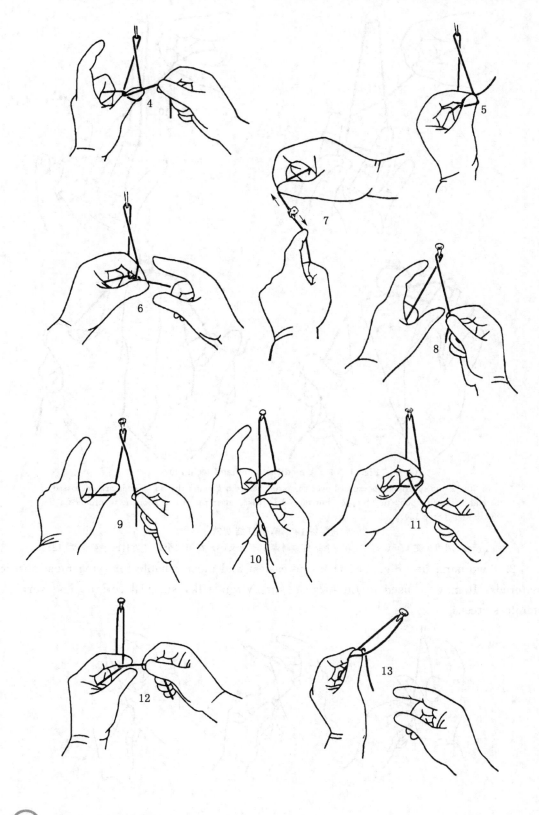

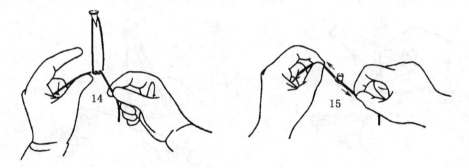

Fig. 1-15   Two-hand square knot

Suture ends are uncrossed as Step 1 begins. Hands must cross at the end of the first loop tie (Step 7) to produce a flat knot. Hands are not crossed at the end of the second loop tie (Step 15).

图 1-15   双手打结法

如 1 所示,两线头不交叉开始打结,第一个结打紧时两手要交叉(7);在第二个结打紧时两手不交叉(15)。

3. Instrument tie: Long end of a strand held between thumb and index finger of left hand. Loop formed by placing needleholder. Needleholder in right hand grasps short end of the strand and make the first simple knot (Fig. 1-16). The instrument tie is useful when one or both ends of the suture material are short.

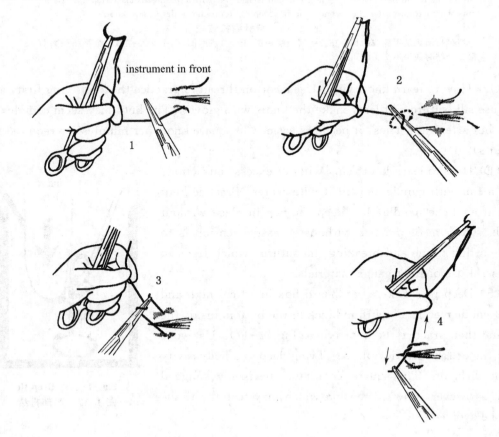

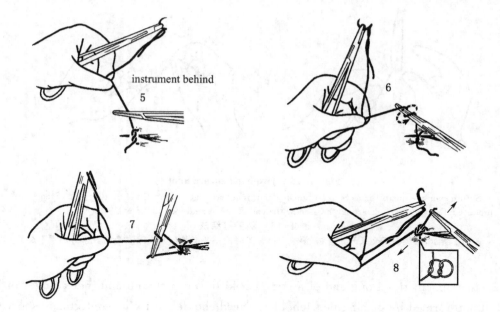

instrument behind

Fig. 1-16 Needleholder tie
The instrument tie begins with either single (illustrated) or double looping of the long end of the suture about the needleholder. The first loop is laid flat with crossing hands (Step 4). Hands must be uncrossed after the second loop tie (Step 8) to produce a flat square knot.

图 1-16 持针钳打结法
器械打结法是用缝线的长头在持针器上绕一圈(图示)或两圈,两手交叉打第一个平结(4);打第二个结时两手不交叉(8)。

(D) How to learn knot tying: Use a cotton thread to practice the knot tying first, and then use silk suture. At last, make the knots with gloves. The knot may seem complex at first, but after a few tries, it becomes easier (30 square knots per minutes are required for students).

(E) How to learn knot tying without excessive traction: Take a cup with handle and fill it with water. Practice knot tying around the handle, but keep the cup in place without splash. The aim of practice without excessive tension is to avoid cutting tissue and breaking the suture, which leads to successful use of finer gauge materials.

(F) Deep tie: Take a cardboard box in 10 cm high and 8~10 cm diameter. Fix a thumbtack in the bottom inside the box and then practice the knot tying (Fig. 1-17). Use your index finger for deep tie, please! Tying deep in a body cavity can be difficult. The square knot must be firmly snugged down. However, upward tension which may tear the tissue must be avoided.

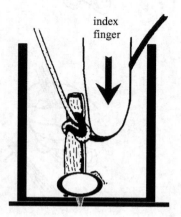

index finger

Fig. 1-17 Deep tie
图 1-17 深部打结

实习一 外科无菌技术操作和打结法

【目的和要求】

1. 能正确区别卫生、灭菌、有菌和无菌概念。

2. 能理解无菌技术操作的原理,并能按照无菌规则进行外科无菌技术操作,包括手臂消毒法(洗手)、穿手术衣和戴手套、手术区皮肤消毒和铺无菌巾、单,以及手术进行中的无菌原则等。

3. 熟练地掌握正确的打结法。

【实习程序】

1. 全班分为两个大组:一组进行外科无菌技术操作,另一组练习打结,2小时后对换。

2. 两大组实习前,分别由教师先行示教,然后学生进行练习。

【实习项目】

一、外科无菌技术操作

(一)手术人员的术前准备

1. 更衣等准备

(1)换手术室专用鞋。

(2)戴好手术帽/兜帽和口罩。

(3)换穿手术室洗手用衣、裤。

(4)勿留长指甲,必要时修剪之。

2. 手臂消毒

大多数手术部位感染的病原菌是病人或手术人员皮肤上正常存在的细菌,主要是金黄色葡萄球菌。正常皮肤的细菌可分为表浅暂驻菌和深藏在汗腺、皮脂腺和毛囊内的常驻菌两种(图1-1)。暂驻菌用肥皂和水很容易洗掉,但常驻菌用外科皮肤杀菌剂也不能完全杀灭。术前用杀菌剂的目的一方面是将皮肤常驻菌的数量降至最低。戴上手套后,皮肤和手套之间的湿润环境有利于细菌的繁殖,其细菌量可以在手术结束时达到洗手前的量。可见外科洗手还远不能令人满意。

(1)肥皂刷手法

① 用普通肥皂将手、前臂、肘和上臂先洗一遍,**肥皂洗手要求两手反复揉搓**,如此可以去除皮肤上的有机和无机物。然后,用流水彻底漂洗手臂。

② 用灭菌毛刷蘸足灭菌肥皂液(或肥皂)刷洗双手至肘上 10 cm,刷时要求用力适度。过度的擦刷会划伤皮肤,反而有利于细菌生长。**刷手时最易疏忽手指尖、指蹼、腕部尺侧和**

肘窝部,须特别注意。

先将手指并拢刷指尖,再由拇指的桡侧起,依次到背侧、尺侧。顺序刷完五指,然后再刷手掌和手背,最后是前臂和肘上等处(图1-2)。绝不能逆着顺序倒回去刷已经刷过的部位。

③ 每刷洗一遍后用流水(自来水)冲洗一次,然后换新刷重复刷洗,共3次,每次3分钟。冲洗时,肘部应弯曲在下(低位),手部向上(高位),防止上臂水流向手部(图1-2-4)。注意勿在肘后部皮肤上遗留肥皂泡沫。

也可以用计次的方法洗手,先刷手指尖和手各20次(一个来回组合为1次),然后换刷另一个手的手指。手臂的四面各10次。

洗过的手不允许碰触水槽、水龙头和洗手衣。还要避免流水溅湿洗手衣。

即使在如今的条件下,在每天的第一例手术前,或在脏手术后,都必须对双手和前臂做彻底洗刷至少5分钟;在之后的每例手术前,至少洗刷3分钟。

④ 用毛巾揩手和臂(图1-2-5):取折叠的无菌毛巾一块,两手将毛巾沿长轴展开,用毛巾的一端揩一侧手臂,从手向上依次揩干手和前臂,揩到肘部后不得返回再揩手部;然后用毛巾的另一端揩另一侧手臂。注意握毛巾的手不要触到已揩过的一端。如果是小毛巾,可以取两块,一块揩一侧手臂。同时还应注意毛巾不要触到未洗刷过的皮肤,以免污染已洗过的区域。将揩过的毛巾丢在洗涤篮内。

⑤ 泡手:将双手和前臂包括肘以上6 cm以内的部分浸在1:1 000苯扎溴铵(新洁尔灭)或75%酒精溶液内5分钟,可以使细菌数迅速减少,浸泡时两手在桶内用纱布揉搓效果更好。伸入和离开浸泡桶时,注意手和前臂不要碰触桶边。

⑥ 手泡好离开浸泡桶后,立即将双手上举呈拱手姿势,将手和上臂的酒精或新洁尔灭滴入桶内。

(2)杀菌剂洗手法:用流水和肥皂先把手和前臂彻底洗一遍,达肘上10厘米,两手相互揉搓1分钟。然后,用流水彻底洗去手臂上的肥皂泡。

用刷子蘸皮肤杀菌剂洗刷手和前臂,聚维酮碘或氯己定要求洗刷3分钟,含乙醇洗手剂则要求洗刷60秒。然后,两手相互揉搓片刻,要注意指蹼和指背的揉搓,不留缝隙。流水彻底洗去手臂上的杀菌剂。

保持屈肘位使手高于肘部,使手臂的水滴入水槽内。径直步入手术间,用背部或髋部推开手术间的门后入内。然后,将手揩干,着手穿衣和戴手套。

3. 穿无菌手术衣和戴无菌手套

(1)穿无菌手术衣:像日常的衣服一样,手术衣也有两个面:反面(内里)可以与手和未灭菌的洗手衣接触,正面是无菌的。手术衣的折叠规则是将衣服的反面露在外面,把衣服的正面折在里面,如此,洗过的手就可以直接抓取手术衣。

取出无菌手术衣,走到较空的地方。通过衣领辨认衣服的上下。提住衣服的内面衣肩处,松开手术衣,勿让手术衣碰及地面。找到袖管开口,两手伸展同时插入袖管,然后屈肘、两臂夹住衣服,由巡回护士在背后拉衣服的肩内面协助穿衣、系好颈部和背部的衣带。最后两手交叉拿住腰带中段向后递,由巡回护士系紧(图1-3)。注意:拿腰带时应稍弯腰,使腰带悬空,以免手触到手术衣的正面。

(2)开放式戴手套法:开放式戴手套用于不穿无菌手术衣时的无菌操作,如:插导尿管和病人皮肤消毒。开放式戴手套前不需要刷手,但要洗手。

手套也有两个面：内面和外面。在用手接触前，这两面都是无菌的。在戴手套过程中，内面就不再无菌了。因此，**戴手套时只允许手接触内面，皮肤不得触及手套外面**。外科手套的折叠规定手套腕部的内侧面应翻转向外，刷过的裸手可以接触该翻转部。

打开手套的纸包装袋（一般是由巡回护士递上来的灭菌内包装），观察手套，将手套的位置调至掌面向上、拇指朝外。用一手捏住一只手套掌侧的翻转口，为对侧手戴上，该手套的翻转部暂时不动。

用已戴手套的手伸入另一只手套的翻转部之内，将手套托起，为未戴手套的手戴上，注意手套的外面不能触到皮肤；此过程中已戴手套的拇指不要接触手套的内面或皮肤（图1-4）。

最后将袖口折好，塞于手套内。手术前，用无菌水冲净手套外面的滑石粉。

（3）封闭式戴手套法：把手和手指放在衣袖内，不要露出来，注意手的方位。

左手掌朝上，将左手套放在左手掌上，掌对掌，手套的指尖对着肘部。在衣袖内左拇指捏住手套的下翻转缘。右拇指抓住手套的上翻转缘套住左袖口，继续保持手套"掌对掌"的位置。然后，展开手套的翻转部分使之完全套住衣袖，戴好手套。同法戴右手套。裸手不能接触衣服的袖口缘，也不能接触手套的外面（图1-5）。

（4）为他人戴手套法：第一位戴好手套的人，可以按照图1-6所示为之后的、穿好手术衣的手术人员戴手套。

（5）手套和手术衣的脱法

① 术中更换手套的方法：术中如果手套有破损或被污染，就需要更换。用对侧手抓住手套袖口部的外面将手套下拖至手掌处，手套不要触到皮肤，同法将另一只手的手套翻转、脱去（图1-7）。最后，将已经脱去手套的手插入手套与手掌皮肤之间把剩下的一只手套翻转脱去，使后脱的手套内有两只手套。

② 术中更换手术衣和手套的方法：如果术中污染，需要更换手术衣和手套时，可按下法进行。先请巡回护士解开后面的衣带，再面对巡回护士，但要保持一定距离，让她帮你脱去手术衣，然后展开你的手臂手心向上，让她帮你脱手套。必要时再刷手，最后重新穿消毒手术衣和戴手套。

③ 手术结束时手术衣和手套的脱法：先由巡回护士帮你解开衣服后面的带子，你自己用手抓住手术衣的肩部将手术衣翻转脱下。然后，按"手套—手套接触、皮肤—皮肤接触"的脱手套法脱手套。

（二）手术区的准备

1. 手术区皮肤消毒

（1）巡回护士应提前去动物房取兔，麻醉后即负责将手术区毛发剃除。人体手术一般不需要剃除毛发，若毛发影响手术，应在手术前即刻剃除，最好用电剪将毛发剪短，有条件时，也可以用脱毛霜。

（2）皮肤消毒由第一助手在洗手后、未穿手术衣和戴手套前进行。

（3）传统的皮肤消毒一般多用3%碘酊及75%酒精，其范围在人体要包括手术切口以外20 cm。先用碘酊涂擦一遍，待碘酊稍干后再用酒精涂擦脱碘2～3次。

酒精杀菌的机理是使细胞干燥，因此，含酒精的消毒剂，尤其是碘酒，不宜用于阴道、直肠黏膜、小儿皮肤、会阴、阴囊等部位皮肤都不能耐受碘酊的刺激，宜用刺激性小的消毒溶液,如 0.5% 碘伏和氯己定等消毒。皮肤对碘过敏者也不宜用碘酊消毒。皮肤的消毒效果取决于物理和化学两方面,因此,**消毒时纱球应在皮肤上做充分地揉擦**。如此反复消毒三次,至少 5 分钟。

(4) 皮肤消毒应由中心部开始,从中央逐渐向外周涂擦,已触及周围皮肤的纱布不可返回中心部。

传统的腹部消毒是用碘伏纱球从上至下纵向进行,先切口中央,后两侧。第二次消毒的范围稍小于第一次,第三次小于第二次(图 1-8)。也可以由外围向内呈环形消毒(图 1-9)。

感染病灶或肛门部消毒,要先用一块浸满消毒液的纱球覆盖在感染部位,由外围向内呈环形消毒,逐渐达污染区。接触污染区后的纱球应随即丢弃。

2. 铺无菌巾、单

皮肤消毒完毕后,需要铺无菌外科方巾和手术单,仅暴露手术部位,创建无菌区。

(1) 铺无菌巾、单是第一助手的工作,一般在穿好手术衣、戴上手套后进行。手术护士,将无菌方巾的 1/4 处折为双层递给第一助手进行铺巾,每次递一块。递无菌方巾时,护士抓住方巾的两端,第一助手抓方巾的内侧。

(2) 铺巾:铺巾时,折叠部分朝下铺盖,防止手套被污染。每块方巾距切口 2～3 cm。铺盖的顺序是:本侧、下方、上方、对侧。然后用巾钳在四角夹好。无菌方巾在铺盖时不可触及任何未灭菌的物品,铺盖后准许自手术区向外移,但不可向内移。铺巾者的两手不要交叉。

倘若铺巾者未穿无菌手术衣,则方巾的铺盖顺序是下方、对侧、上方、本侧。

最后在切口上贴切口膜。切口膜也可以在铺完手术单后贴。

(3) 铺无菌手术单:在第一助手穿上手术衣和戴好手套后,由第一助手和手术护士合作铺手术单。手术单上的特定位置通常有大小不等的开孔(窗)。由于手术的部位和种类各异,因此,开窗手术单有多种。剖腹单是指用于腹部手术的手术单。手术单的折叠方式要求在折叠后窗位于中央。铺剖腹单时要辨认其上、下标记。将剖腹单中心孔对准切口部,向两侧铺开时先铺本侧,后铺对侧,然后先向上方、后向下方展开剖腹单。展开剖腹单时,应抓住剖腹单边将手卷在剖腹单里面,以免手碰脏。上方(头端)盖过麻醉头架,两侧和足端下垂至手术台边缘下 31～40 cm。

(4) 铺无菌巾、单时除操作者外,其他人都应远离,以防弄脏。在铺单完毕前,操作者与手术台应保持适当距离,以免手术衣碰脏。手术单铺定后,不允许再挪动,若手术单铺置欠满意,可以另加手术单。

(三)小无菌包裹的打开

先检查包裹布有无破损。用手打开外层包布,调整包裹的方向。用灭菌卵圆钳打开内层包布,把包布上叶打开翻向对侧,两个侧叶翻向两侧,最后将下叶翻向本侧。

(四)手术进行中的无菌原则

无菌野对外科来说至关重要,只有无菌物品和人员才能接触无菌野。为了在手术进行中保持无菌,参加手术的人员必须自觉地遵守下列规则:

1. 无菌野应该在视野之内。发现自己或别人违反无菌原则时，应立即指出并报告洗手护士。**"有疑问时，按污染处理"**。如无菌区可疑碰污，经其他人员提出时，不得强辩、解释，否则，他（她）就没有资格在手术室工作或学习。在手术室的无菌术字典上，没有"妥协"二字。

2. 手术单铺完后，无菌区的范围是前胸自腰部或手术台至胸中部、手套、衣袖从肘上5厘米至袖口、手术台面和器械台，手术衣的背部、肩部和腰部以下均为有菌区，因此，要注意肘部不碰及手术台旁的参观人员，手不能插入腋下（图1-10）。

手术单两边的下垂部分，手术台头架以外和器械台以外的布单都被认为是有菌区。任何超出手术台缘的物品都应看作是有菌的。如果手术人员需要足凳，足凳应该在手术人员站位前放置，避免在手术过程中自下向上移动，造成无菌野污染、缩小。有菌人员或物品应距无菌区30 cm以上。

取递无菌器械时不能越过有菌区域，如不应从无菌人员的头上越过或背后传送。有菌人员也不能越过无菌区取物。

3. 整个手术过程中，无菌人员应该紧靠手术台站立，面朝无菌区，尽可能少移动。无菌人员更换位置时必须面向无菌的手术台或器械桌，然后背对背地转360°交换位置（图1-11）。无菌人员在移动中应该背对有菌的人员或物品。

4. 布类一经潮湿即可能因毛细现象而伴有细菌通过，无菌隔离即被破坏，最好用不透水的带黏性边的无菌巾覆盖。如衣袖被汗水浸湿，应更换。

5. 手套有破孔，在病人安全允许的情况下应立即更换。有研究表明，针眼大的破孔，在20分钟内可有数以万计的细菌通过。

6. 接触过皮肤的器械（如手术刀）不能再用。切开空腔脏器（如胃肠、胆道）前或在其他污染源开放前，应该用纱布或薄膜把周围的正常器官组织隔开、保护起来，要另外打开一套器械，把接触清洁部位的器械与接触污染区域的器械分开。有关部分操作完毕后，这些污染的器械即不应再用，医生要重新换衣服和手套才能用无菌器械操作。

7. 应尽可能地减少进出手术室的人流和手术室内的谈话。手术中应避免面对无菌区咳嗽或打喷嚏，不得已时头可转向身后。

8. 如手术需暂停（如等待病理冰冻切片报告），切口应用无菌巾覆盖。病人躁动时须注意约束病人手臂，使之不致进入手术区内。手术完毕缝合切口前，切口两旁皮肤以酒精涂擦一遍。

9. 两台手术同时进行时，不应互相拿用器械和用品。

10. 由钳夹或干燥造成的损伤组织愈合缓慢，并且容易发生感染，因此，手术中对组织操作轻柔、彻底止血、尽可能地减少失活组织和异物（缝线、焦痂）可以降低感染发生率。结扎止血时，尽可能少带周围组织。

二、打结法

1. 手术中经常需要结扎止血，组织缝合后也要打结使其对合，因此，正确的结扎是外科的基本功之一。结打得牢固，可以防止线结松动、滑脱。线结滑脱可引起出血或者缝合的组织裂开，给病人带来痛苦，甚至危及生命。

线结总是一个缝合的最弱点。打结时,线两端的用力要相同,方向相反,"三点(线两端和线结)成一线"。打结的速度不要太快,以免成结不满意。

三重结常用于皮肤缝合。从结的牢固性来看,影响线结数的主要因素是材料和工艺。由于单股缝线的表面摩擦力小,因此线结比多股缝合材料容易滑脱。为了防止单股缝线线结的滑脱,通常需要打多重结,形成一个"大结",组织反应也随之增大。

2. 外科基本线结

(1) 方结:是手术中常用的一种打结法,结扎后极为牢固,可用于多种材质缝线的打结,包括丝线。

注意:结口的交叉要对正确,第一单结和第二单结方向相反(图1-12)。两个结打成同一方向就形成假结(图1-12),假结在有张力时很容易滑脱,外科手术中不能用假结。拉紧线时,两手用力要均匀,两手一紧一松就容易形成滑结(图1-12)。

(2) 三重结:就是在打成方结之后,再重复第一单结(图1-12),使结扣更牢固,主要用于合成缝线的打结。

(3) 外科结:打第一结时绕两次,摩擦面比较大,再打第二结时不易滑脱(图1-12)。

3. 打结的方法

(1) 单手打结:一般用右手打结(图1-13),左利者可以通过镜子练习打结。如果在打第二个半结时,食指使用有困难者,可以按照图1-14的变式练习打结。

(2) 双手打结:双手打结很简单,成结可靠,可用大多数材质的缝线,如外科肠线、丝线、外科棉线和外科不锈钢丝(图1-15)。

(3) 器械打结:使用持针钳,绕长线一周,钳夹短线进行打结(图1-16)。持针钳打结一般用于线短时。

4. 学习打结 学会细绳打结后,改用细丝线连续打结,最后,戴上手套再练习打结。开始练打结可能有些困难,以后可以练到不假思索、迅速自如地打成正确的结扣(一般要求每分钟打方结30个)。

5. 学习轻柔打结 取一只有把茶杯,将茶杯中装满水,在茶杯把上练习打结,要求杯子在桌上不移动,水不外溢。轻柔打结的目的是避免组织撕裂和缝线断裂,允许用细线。

6. 深部打结 选一个口径约8~10 cm、高10 cm的纸盒,在其底部按一枚图钉固定缝线,练习打结(图1-17)。深部打结,要用食指!体腔手术时常需要使用深部打结。深部打结要求结打得牢固舒展,避免用上提力撕扯组织。

Session 2　Basic surgical instruments identifying and instrumentation & Common suture methods

【Goals & requirements】

1. Be familiar with common surgical instruments and correct holding.

2. Demonstrate methods of suture.

【Progress schedule】

1. Students will learn identifying common surgical instruments and their correct holding.

2. Educator will demonstrate the techniques of suture first，and then students will be asked to follow step by step. Suture techniques will be practiced on suture training board covered with cloth material.

【Topics of this session】

A. Introduction to basic surgical instruments

See Fig. 2-1 to Fig. 2-6.

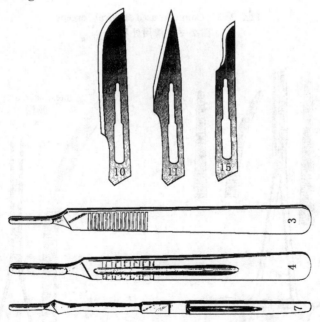

Fig. 2-1　Scalpel blades and scalpel handles
图 2-1　刀和刀柄

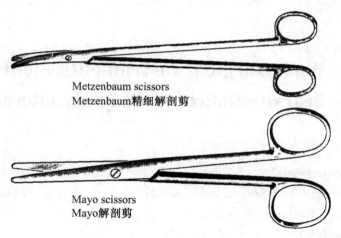

Fig. 2-2　Common used surgical scissors

图 2-2　常用手术剪

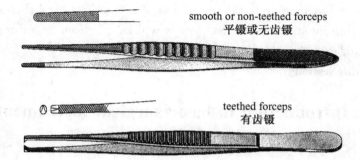

Fig. 2-3　Common used surgical forceps

图 2-3　常用外科镊

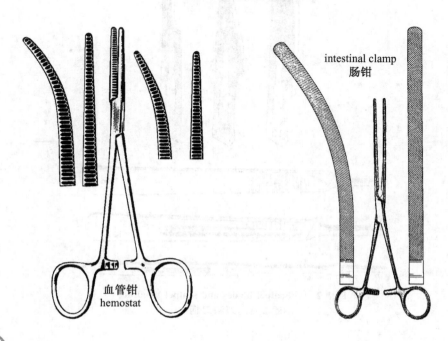

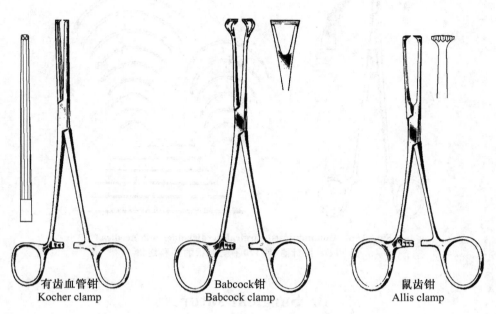

有齿血管钳
Kocher clamp

Babcock钳
Babcock clamp

鼠齿钳
Allis clamp

Fig. 2-4　Common used surgical clamps
图 2-4　常用外科钳

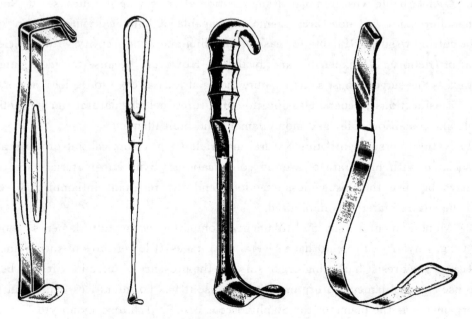

Fig. 2-5　Common used surgical retractors
图 2-5　常用外科拉钩(牵开器)

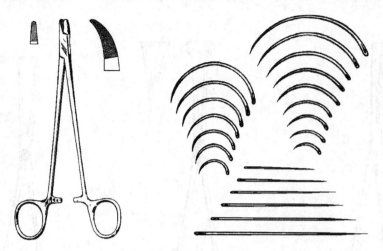

Fig. 2-6　Common used surgical needleholder and needles
图 2-6　持针器（钳）和不同形状的外科缝针

B.　Surgical sutures

1. An ideal suture material should be: ①Sterile, minimally reactive in tissue and not predisposed to bacterial growth. ②All-purpose, composed of material which could be used in any surgical procedure. ③Able to maintain adequate tensile strength until its purpose is served. ④Absorbable with minimal tissue reaction after serving its purpose. ⑤Noncapillary, nonallergenic, and non-carcinogenic. ⑥Capable of holding securely when knotted without cutting tissue. ⑦Pliable for ease of handling and knot security with sufficient coefficient of friction. ⑧Inexpensive and available. However, because the ideal suture does not yet exist, the surgeon must select a suture that is at least as close to the ideal as possible.

2. Classifications. General classification of sutures includes natural and synthetic, absorbable and nonabsorbable, and monofilament and multifilament.

(1) Natural versus synthetic: Natural materials (e. g. , surgical gut or surgical silk) are associated with high rate of wound complications. Synthetic materials are popular these days because they cause less reaction, and the resultant inflammatory reaction around the suture material is minimized.

(2) Monofilament versus multifilament: Comparing with multifilaments, monofilaments (e. g. , nylon or Prolene) have several advantages: ①lower rates of suture line infection because they resist harboring organisms. In the presence of infection, it may be desirable to use a monofilament suture material because it has no interstices which can harbor microorganisms as the diameter for Staphylocccus is $0.7 \sim 1.2 \ \mu m$, monocyte $15 \sim 20 \ \mu m$ and neutrophile granulocyte $12 \sim 15 \ \mu m$. ②less traumatic, since they glide through tissues with less friction, and ③tension suture effects (pulley block mechanism), a continuous suture derives its strength from tension distributed evenly along the full length of the su-

ture strand because of low friction of monofilaments. But monofilaments are susceptible to instrumentation damage and somewhat stiff to handle. Therefore, extra throws are required to secure knots in place. Multifilament (braided) sutures (e. g. , silk or Vicryl) are traumatic, which works in the same way as **a wire saw** as it is drawn through tissues (Fig. 2-14) and, experimentally at least, are associated with greater inflammation and activation of collagenases than monofilament material (e. g. , PDS, Prolene).

(3) Absorbable versus nonabsorbable: Absorption can take from a week to several months depending on material. Any suture that will be buried in tissues should be either absorbable or monofilament (non-absorbable braided suture is irritating and can harbor bacteria).

(4) Gauge for synthetic materials: The common used sizes of suture are 000 (3-0), 00 (2-0), 0, 1 and 2. The diameter of the suture or the thickness of the strand determines its numerical size (Fig. 2-1).

Table 2-1　Gauge for synthetic sutures

Chinese size	USP[1] size	EP[2] size	Diameter (mm)	
			min.	max.
	8-0	0. 4	0. 040	0. 049
	7-0	0. 5	0. 050	0. 069
	6-0	0. 7	0. 070	0. 099
3-0	5-0	1. 0	0. 100	0. 149
0	4-0	1. 5	0. 150	0. 199
1	3-0	2. 0	0. 200	0. 249
4	2-0	3. 0	0. 300	0. 339
7	0	3. 5	0. 350	0. 399
10	1	4	0. 400	0. 499
	2	5	0. 500	0. 599
	3, 4	6	0. 600	0. 699
	5	7	0. 700	0. 799

[1] USP (United States Pharmacopoeia). [2] EP (European Pharmacopoeia). EP is equal to metric.

C. Methods of holding surgical instruments

1. Scalpel: The common surgical scalpel is used for cutting tissue. There are different shapes and size of scalpel blades available. A scalpel blade is detachable from the knife handle. For loading the blade on a scalpel handle, hold the scalpel in your left hand with the hub of the handle away from you and upward. Grasp the tip end and blunt side of a new blade with a hemostat and slide the blade onto the handle. For dismounting the blade

from the handle，hold the scalpel in the same way. Grasp the proximal end of the blade with a hemostat，lift the posterior edge of the blade to clear the hub of the handle and free it by pushing it up over the end of the handle (Fig. 2-7). There are five ways of holding scalpel (Fig. 2-8)：

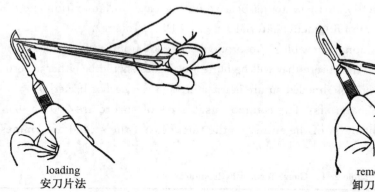

loading
安刀片法

removal
卸刀片法

Fig. 2-7 Methods of mounting and removing knife blades
图 2-7 手术刀装、卸法

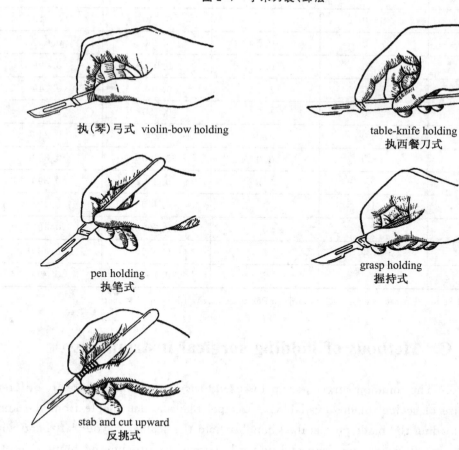

执(琴)弓式 violin-bow holding

table-knife holding
执西餐刀式

pen holding
执笔式

grasp holding
握持式

stab and cut upward
反挑式

Fig. 2-8 Methods of holding the scalpel
图 2-8 五种常用执刀方式

(1) Table-knife holding：This is the most commonly used holding method of scalpel, especially for long incision, e. g. , thoracic or abdominal incision. The shaft of scalpel is grasped between the thumb and the third and fourth fingers with the index finger placed over the back of the blade. The whole upper extremity moves with cutting.

(2) Violin-bow holding：The scalpel is grasped as the table-knife holding, but the index finger is rested in front of the middle finger.

(3) Pencil holding：If you want to make short incision or to cut more gently, e. g. , dissecting blood vessel or nerve, hold it like a pen to facilitate control. A small blade allows you to make precise turns. The movement is limited to the fingers and wrist.

(4) Grasp holding：The scalpel is grasped with the shaft of the scalpel in the palm of your hand when you need force to make a big bold cut, e. g. , amputation.

(5) Stab and cut upward：Hold the scalpel as if it was a pencil but the cutting edge is upward to avoid injury of deep structure. Stab the point of a No. 11 blade into an abscess and then sweep it upwards in an arc.

2. Surgical scissors：There are two kinds of surgical scissors, one is tissue scissors for dissection or cutting tissue and the other is suture scissors for cutting suture, gauze and draining tubes. Use straight scissors near the surface and curved ones deeper inside. The method for holding the scissors is to place the thumb and ring finger slightly into the instrument's rings (Fig. 2-9). This allows you to pronate and supinate and to open and close the blades of the scissors. Avoid inserting your fingers far into the rings of the instrument, since this will tie up your fingers and impede your mobility.

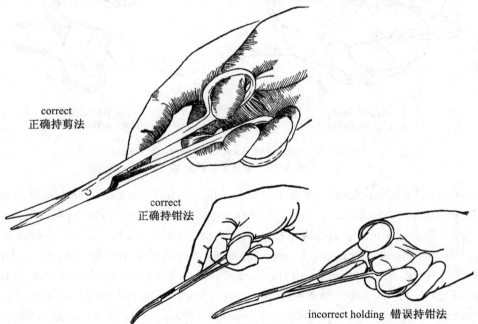

correct
正确持剪法

correct
正确持钳法

incorrect holding 错误持钳法

Fig. 2-9   Method of holding the surgical scissors or clamps
图 2-9   执手术剪(钳)姿势

Tissue scissors are used for cutting tissue, e. g., cutting the ligated vessel. You can also use scissors for blunt dissection by pushing their blades into tissues and then opening them. This will open the tissues along their natural planes, and push important structures, such as nerves and blood vessels, out of the way. This is the "push and spread" technique.

3. Common used surgical clamps: These instruments have numberous variations. It may be straight or curved jaws, full teeth or half teeth, toothed or smooth (noncrushing), and long, middle or small size. Clamps are used to compress the walls of vessels together and also for grasping tissue. Most commonly used is the hemostat. Straight hemostats are used near the surface or subcutaneous hemostasis and curved ones deeper inside, half toothed for abdominal wall and full toothed for intraabdomen, and mosquito hemostat (the smallest one) for fine dissection and hemostasis.

Hemostatic clamps are the main means of grasping vessel or bleeding point and establishing hemostasis during surgery. They may also be used for dissection, holding suture, and grasping and drawing needle. Method of holding the hemostats is the same as holding surgical scissors (Fig. 2-9). Left and right hands have the same method to lock the hemostat, but different in unlocking it (Fig. 2-10): right thumb and ring finger are slightly placed into the instrument's rings for opening a hemostat, but left thumb and index finger hold one instrument's ring away from you when left middle finger push the other ring.

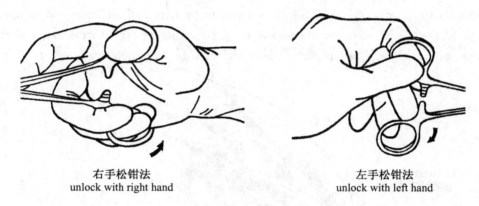

右手松钳法
unlock with right hand

左手松钳法
unlock with left hand

Fig. 2-10 Method of releasing the surgical clamps
图 2-10 松血管钳的姿势

4. Surgical needleholder(needle driver) (Fig. 2-6): Surgical needleholder may be straight or angled. The latter are useful when working at a depth or where there is a space constraint. The size of the needleholder must correspond to the size of needle it must grasp. Needles should be gripped at approximately one-third of the distance from the blunt end of the needle, at right angles to the needle holder, proximal to the tip and at the first ratchet (Fig. 2-11). There are several techniques for holding the needle holder. The most common method is the same as holding a scissors (Fig. 2-9). Some surgeons do not put their fingers into the rings at all and simply grasp the rings and body of the needleholder in the palm of their hand (Fig. 2-12). Needleholder can also be used to make tie (Fig. 1-16).

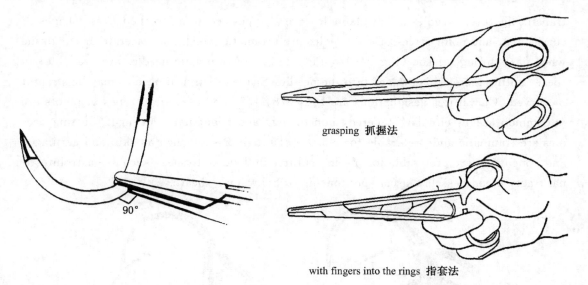

grasping 抓握法

with fingers into the rings 指套法

Fig. 2-11   Arm a needleholder properly
图 2-11   持针钳夹针的位置

Fig. 2-12   Method of holding needleholder
（needle driver）
图 2-12   执持针钳姿势

5. Surgical forceps: These may be toothed or non-toothed and are used for holding tissue during dissection or suturing. Toothed forceps are preferable for grasping tough tissue, such as skin, fascia and tendon, and the non-toothed are preferable for clamping delicate tissues, such as blood vessels, nerves or mucosa. They are held between the thumb and the middle and index fingers of either hand with exerting adequate pressure to hold tissue (Fig. 2-13).

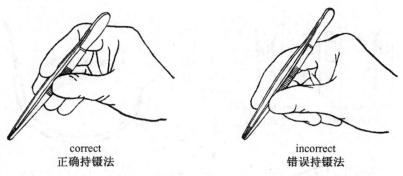

correct
正确持镊法

incorrect
错误持镊法

Fig. 2-13   Method of holding the forceps
图 2-13   执手术镊（钳）的姿势

6. Retractor: As the surgical wound is made deeper, a retractor is required to move tissue layers and structures away from the focal point of the operation and to create exposure. There are two major types of retractors: hand-held and self-retaining. There are numerous variations (shape and size) of retractors. A gauze sponge should be placed between the retractor and tissues at the edge of the wound or the vital structure, e. g. , liver.

7. Surgical needles: Needles are used to introduce suture for tissue approximate or

transfix ligature. Needles are available in several types according to their eyes, shapes or curvatures, and point styles. Eyed needles are traumatic which may lacerate or cut tissue when pass through tissue (Fig. 2-14, Fig. 2-15). Atraumatic needles are available; in these, suture material is swaged into the needle. Shape of surgical needles may be straight or curved. Curvatures designations are 1/4, 3/8, 1/2, and 5/8. Two types of points are in common usage: circular (tapered, noncutting) and triangular (cutting). Cutting needles are traumatic and preferable for closure of tough tissue, such as skin and cartilage, and noncutting are preferable for placing sutures in delicate tissues, such as gastrointestinal tract, blood vessels, fascia, peritoneum or Schwann's sheath.

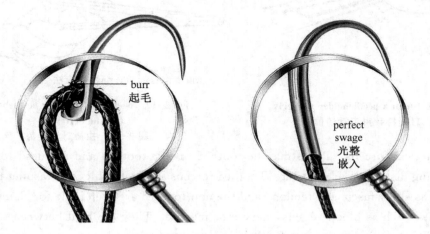

Fig. 2-14　Eyed needles and multifilament suture are traumatic

图 2-14　有针眼缝针和多股缝线可造成损伤

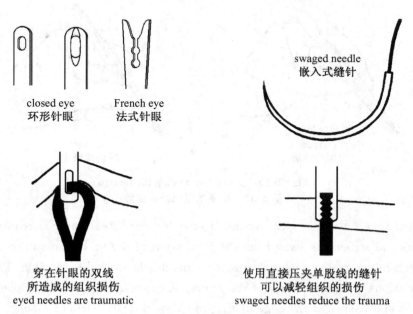

closed eye
环形针眼

French eye
法式针眼

swaged needle
嵌入式缝针

穿在针眼的双线
所造成的组织损伤
eyed needles are traumatic

使用直接压夹单股线的缝针
可以减轻组织的损伤
swaged needles reduce the trauma

Fig. 2-15　Eyed (traumatic) needles and atraumatic needles

图 2-15　有损伤和无损伤缝针

8. Surgical instruments passing: Instruments should be passed in a positive and decisive manner. When an instrument is properly passed, the surgeon will know he has it and will not have to move his eyes from operative field (Fig. 2-16). The scrub nurse and the assistants should know what he wants by his signals. When he extends his hand the instrument should be slapped firmly into his palm, in proper position for use when he closes his hand on it. All instruments are passed in their closed (locked) position unless the surgeon requests otherwise.

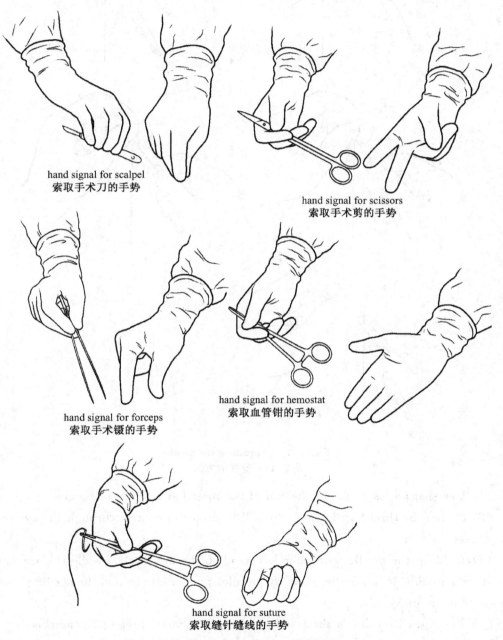

hand signal for scalpel
索取手术刀的手势

hand signal for scissors
索取手术剪的手势

hand signal for forceps
索取手术镊的手势

hand signal for hemostat
索取血管钳的手势

hand signal for suture
索取缝针缝线的手势

Fig. 2-16　Hand signals for surgical instruments
图 2-16　索取手术器械的手势

9. Placing suture in needle (Fig. 2-17):

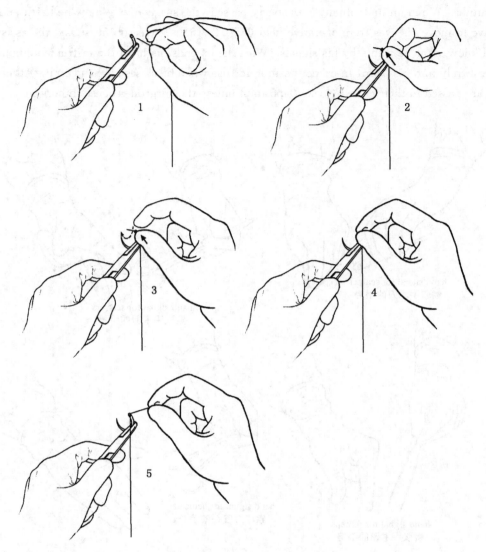

Fig. 2-17 Threading the needle
图 2-17 穿线的方法

（1）Use sharp scissors to cut the end of the thread at a 45 degree angle.

（2）Stiffen the thread with water. It will be easier to control through the eye than a limp thread.

（3）Hold up the needle with your left hand so the eye of the needle is open toward you. If you are unable to see the eye of the needle, place white behind the needle, it makes the eye much more visible.

（4）The right hand holds the last 1 centimeter of your thread perpendicular to your needle. The end of the thread is passed through the eye of the needle. Once you can see some of the thread through the eye, press the thread on the eye with your right thumb to keep the thread in place. This will help keeping the needle from becoming un-threaded as you work. Then, release your right forefinger, use the finger to take the end of the thread which has come through and pull the thread through the eye far enough to create a tail of thread that's 8 to 10 centimeters long.

NOTE: I am right-handed, so the pictures are drawn as a right-handed person threads the needle. If you are left-handed, you may have to reverse my instructions (put the figure in front of a mirror).

D. Surgical sutures

（A）Suturing techniques

Suture variations are numerous. There are three basic techniques: simple appositional, inverting and everting suture, each one of which may be interrupted or continuous. The most important for this training program is simple interrupted suture, "figure of eight" suture, simple running suture and purse string suture.

1. Simple interrupted suture or everting interrupted suture (Fig. 2-18): It is commonly used in skin or subcutaneous tissue closure. Strive to evert the edges and avoid tension on the skin, while approximating the wound edges. Place all knots on the same side. Epidermal skin sutures function for fine alignment of skin edges. **Interrupted sutures are less constrictive than running sutures.**

2. Through-and-through suture or "figure of eight" suture (Fig. 2-19): It is a kind of tension suture used for closing the subcutaneous tissue, fascia or tendon.

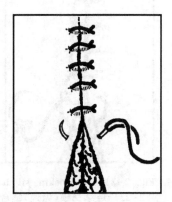

Fig. 2-18   **Simple interrupted suture or everting interrupted suture**
图 2-18   单纯间断缝合

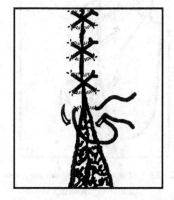

Fig. 2-19   **Through-and-through suture or "figure of eight" suture**
图 2-19   双间断缝合（"8"字形缝合）

3. Interrupted vertical mattress sutures: A vertical mattress suture is an excellent

way of making sure that skin edges are everted. There is a small superficial bite and a large deeper one. This suture can aid in everting the skin edges and is commonly used in body sites where the wound edges tend to invert, such as the posterior neck or wounds that occur on a concave surface or skin of scrotum.

4. Interrupted horizontal mattress sutures (Fig. 2-21): This technique is commonly used for pulling wound edges together over a distance, or as the initial suture to anchor two wound edges (holding sutures).

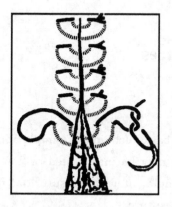

Fig. 2-20　Interrupted vertical mattress suture
图 2-20　间断垂直褥式缝合

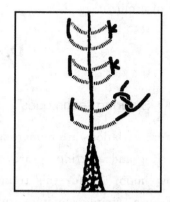

Fig. 2-21　Interrupted horizontal mattress suture
图 2-21　间断水平褥式缝合

5. Simple running suture (Fig. 2-22): It is commonly used in peritoneum closure because it is more watertight.

6. Simple locked running suture or interlocking stitch (Fig. 2-23): This technique is commonly used in gastrointestinal anastomoses, peritoneum closure and anchoring skin graft.

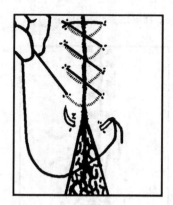

Fig. 2-22　Simple running suture, over
and over running stitch,
continuous suture
图 2-22　单纯连续缝合

Fig. 2-23　Interlocking stitch
图 2-23　连续交锁(毯边)缝合

7. Interrupted inverting seromuscular suture or Lembert suture (Fig. 2-24, Fig. 3-6): A Lembert suture is most commonly used in outer (seromuscular) layer of a gastrointestinal anasto-

mosis.

8. Interrupted horizontal mattress seromuscular inverting suture or Halsted suture (Fig. 2-25): A Halsted suture is commonly used in outer (seromuscular) layer of a gastrointestinal anastomosis.

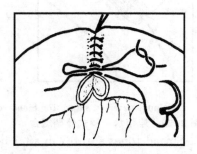

Fig. 2-24 Interrupted inverting seromuscular
suture or Lembert suture
图 2-24 间断浆肌层内翻缝合（Lembert 缝合）

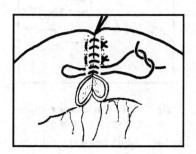

Fig. 2-25 Interrupted horizontal mattress
seromuscular inverting suture or
Halsted suture
图 2-25 间断水平褥式浆肌层内翻缝合
（Halsted 缝合）

9. Continuous inverting seromuscular suture or Cushing suture (Fig. 2-26): This suture method entails similar technique to Connell suture but the submucosa and mucosa layers are not penetrated. A Cushing suture is commonly used in outer (seromuscular) layer of a gastrointestinal anastomosis.

10. Continuous full-layer inverting suture or Connell suture (Fig. 2-27): A Connell suture is commonly used in inner (full) layer of a gastrointestinal anastomosis.

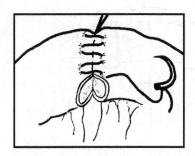

Fig. 2-26 Continuous inverting seromuscular
suture or Cushing suture
图2-26 连续浆肌层内翻缝合（Cushing 缝合）

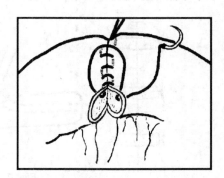

Fig. 2-27 Continuous full-layer inverting
suture or Connell suture
图 2-27 连续全层内翻缝合（Connell 缝合）

11. Purse string suture (Fig. 2-28): A purse string suture is commonly used for the management of the appendix stump.

12. Continuous horizontal mattress everting suture (Fig. 2-29): A continuous horizontal mattress everting suture is commonly used in blood vessel anastomosis.

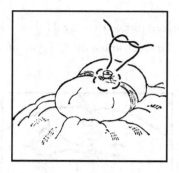

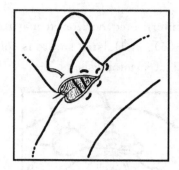

Fig. 2-28　Purse string suture
图 2-28　荷包缝合

Fig. 2-29　Continuous everted suture for blood vessel
图 2-29　连续水平褥式外翻缝合

13. Smead-Jones far-and-near suture (Fig. 2-30): Smead-Jones suture, in a far-near-near-far fashion, is a tension suture and may used to close the abdominal wall.

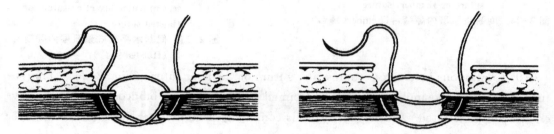

Fig. 2-30　Smead-Jones far-near-near-far suture
图 2-30　"远—近—近—远"缝合(Smead-Jones 缝合)

14. Tension suture (Fig. 2-31):

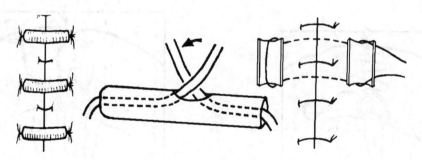

Fig. 2-31　Tension suture
图 2-31　减张缝合(张力缝合)

15. Subcuticular suture (intracutaneous suture) (Fig. 2-32): To minimizing the railroad tract scarring, suturing the subcuticular layer of tough connective tissue will hold the skin edges in close approximation. The surgeon takes short lateral stitches beneath the epithelial layer of skin. If nonabsorbable material is used, one end of the suture strand will protrude from each end of the incision, and the surgeon may tie them together to form a "loop" or knot the ends outside of the incision.

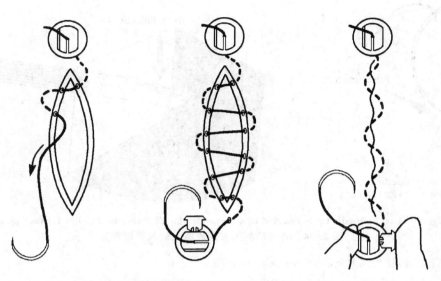

Fig. 2-32   Subcuticular suture or intracutaneous suture
图 2-32   表皮下连续缝合（皮内缝合）

（B）Basic surgical principles of suture

Basic surgical principles of suture is closure without tension, elimination of dead space, and taking the greatest care to ensure that wound edges not only are aligned but also are everted.

1. Ideally the needle driver should be lined up parallel to the proposed suture line (Fig. 2-33). And the needle is rotated and pivoted until the angle of needle insertion into tissue of 80 degrees to 100 degrees (Fig. 2-34).

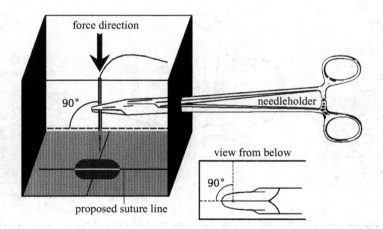

Fig. 2-33   The needleholder should be parallel to the proposed suture line
图 2-33   持针器的轴向应该尽可能与拟缝合线的轴向平行

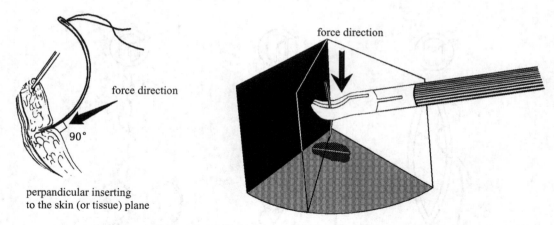

Fig. 2-34　The needle tip is inserted in a perpendicular direction to the skin（tissue）plane

图 2-34　针尖的刺入方向应该与刺入平面垂直

2. Ablate all "dead space" during closure.

3. Accurate tissue apposition. Strive to evert the edges and avoid tension on the skin, while approximating the wound edges （Fig. 2-35）.

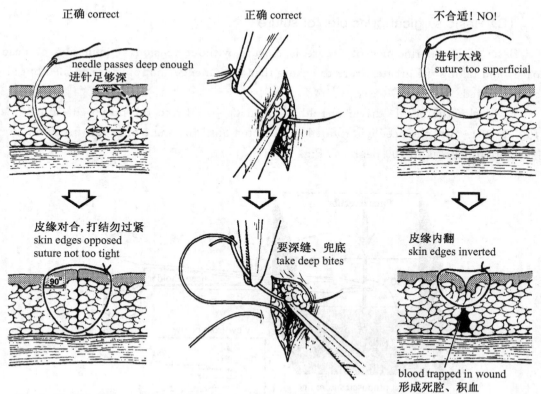

Fig. 2-35　Suturing a wound. The dotted line shows the path of the suture. If "X" is smaller than "Y", the skin edges will be everted. The suture should enter the skin at 90°

图 2-35　伤口的缝合原则　图中的虚线示缝线的径路。如果"X"比"Y"短，创缘就外翻。进针的方向应该与皮肤平面呈 90°

4. Oppose equal amounts of tissue on each side. The needle should exit through the opposite side equidistant to the wound edge and directly opposite the initial insertion.

5. Interrupted sutures are inserted at adequate intervals, taking bites 1 cm from the cut edge and 1 cm apart (Fig. 2-36).

6. Take great care to avoid tension during closure, which will lead to tissue strangulation and necrosis.

7. Bleeding might occur through needle holes when vessel is penetrated. The correct way to manage this situation is to withdraw the needle, especially for eyed needles, and exert outside pressure over any small needle holes to prevent bleeding (Fig. 2-37).

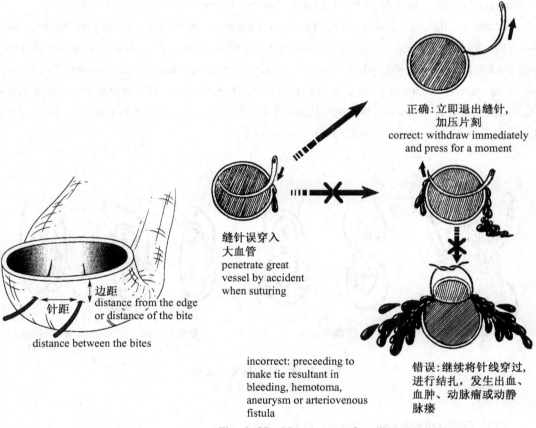

正确:立即退出缝针,
加压片刻
correct: withdraw immediately
and press for a moment

缝针误穿入
大血管
penetrate great
vessel by accident
when suturing

边距
distance from the edge
or distance of the bite

针距

distance between the bites

incorrect: preceeding to
make tie resultant in
bleeding, hemotoma,
aneurysm or arteriovenous
fistula

错误:继续将针线穿过,
进行结扎,发生出血、
血肿、动脉瘤或动静
脉瘘

**Fig. 2-36   Distance of bite and
distance between the
bites**

图 2-36   缝合的边距与针距

**Fig. 2-37   Management of needle hole bleeding
when making a suture**

It is prudent to suture-ligate vessels within the thick, edematous mesentery rather than use simple ligatures that may slip.

图 2-37   缝合遇到血管出血时的处理

在处理增厚、水肿的肠系膜时,最好能对系膜血管进行缝扎,不要做单纯的结扎,以免线结滑脱。

（C）Common methods of securing hemostasis

1. Free tie ligature：The crushing clamp is used to establish hemostasis at the divided ends of blood vessels of all size. Since the clamped tissue will be destroyed，the tip of the clamp should grasp the end of the blood vessel, the tip of the vessel only and not the adjacent tissue. Continued hemostasis is assured if the end of the vessel is tied.

A tie is passed around the vessel at the tip of the hemostat and the first half hitch is set (Fig. 1-13-1). While this is being done，the assistant should hold the clamp in such a way that the tip of the instrument is exposed to the operator. To elevate the tip of the clamp the handle is depressed. After the first half hitch is set，the assistant removes the hemostat；the first half hitch is tightened further before the second is begun.

2. Suture ligature (stick tie or transfixion suture)：Stick tie is placed on an important vessel to avoid slipping. It must be placed back on the vessel sufficiently far to preclude the possibility of one side of the suture slipping over the end of the vessel. "Figure of eight" suture is commonly used in this situation (Fig. 2-38). If atraumatic sutures are available，a suture is passed through the middle of the vessel，and it is tied first around one half of the vessel and then around the entire vessel.

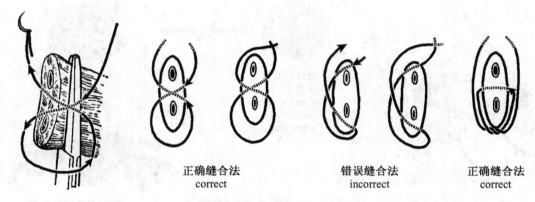

正确缝合法 correct 　　　　错误缝合法 incorrect 　　　　正确缝合法 correct

Fig. 2-38　Making a stick tie
图 2-38　缝合止血法

（D）Cutting sutures

Once the knot has been securely tied，the ends must be cut. Before cutting，make sure both tips of the scissors are visible to avoid inadvertently cutting important tissue beyond the suture. Cutting sutures entails slipping the suture scissors，with tips open (close the scissors most of the way)，lightly down along the suture to the knot，twisting the tip (about 45°) to allow the desired length of tail and cutting the suture (Fig. 2-39).

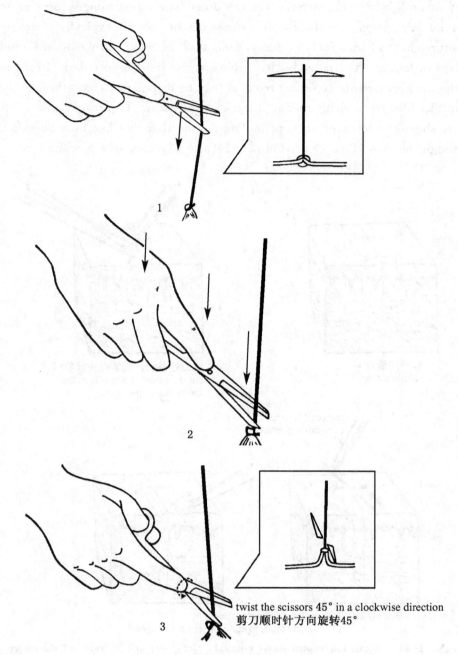

twist the scissors 45° in a clockwise direction
剪刀顺时针方向旋转45°

Fig. 2-39   Method of suture cutting
图 2-39   剪线法

（E）Removing sutures

Only the skin sutures must be removed. These skin sutures should be removed as soon as adequate intrinsic bonding strength is sufficient. Skin sutures left in place too long result in an unsightly track pattern. On the other hand, removing sutures prematurely risks wound dehiscence. Nonabsorbable sutures on the face are typically removed after 5 days. Sutures in the hand, foot, or across areas that are acted on by motion should be left for 14 days or longer. Alternatively, by employing the running intradermal suturing technique, the time constraints of suture removal may be disregarded, and these sutures may be left in place longer without risking a track pattern scar. To prevent risk of infection, the suture should be removed without pulling any portion that has been outside the skin back through the skin (Fig. 2-40, Fig. 2-41)(also reference to Appendix 5).

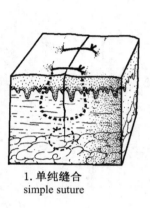

1. 单纯缝合
simple suture

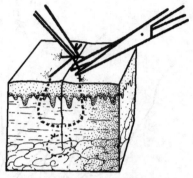

2. 靠线结的一端紧贴皮肤剪线
cut the suture at one side of the knot close to the skin

correct direction
of removing suture

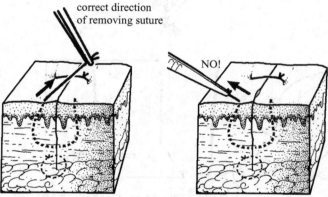

3. 抽线的方向 pull out a suture so that a wound tends to close rather than to open

Fig. 2-40　Simple interrupted suture removal　Grasp one of the "ears" of the suture with a forceps to elevate the suture just enough to slip the tip of a small scissor under the suture in order to cut it. This should be done close to the skin edge in order to minimize the amount of contaminated suture that will be dragged through the stitch path. The suture is then gently removed by pulling with the forceps

图 2-40　单纯缝合线的拆线法　用手术镊夹住并提起线结,以便剪刀尖端能插入缝线内。贴近缝线入皮处剪线,以减少外露的缝线在移除时进入组织内。然后,用镊子按一定方向轻轻拖出剪断的缝线

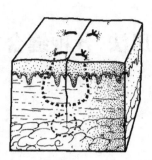

1. 褥式缝合
vertical mattress sutures

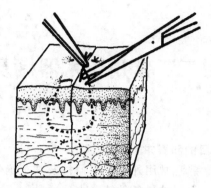

2. 靠线结的一端紧贴皮肤剪线
grasp the knot and cut
one side of the knot

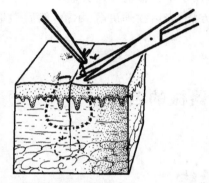

3. 镊子不松动，紧贴皮肤
剪线结的另一端
still hold the knot and cut
the other side of the knot

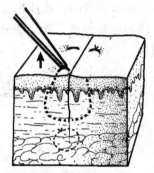

4. 弃线结，镊子夹住切口
另一侧露出的线向上抽
discard the knot, grasp the suture
outside the skin and remove it

Fig. 2-41　Interrupted vertical mattress suture removal
图 2-41　褥式缝合线的拆线法(抓住线结,在线结的两侧各剪一次)

实习二 常用手术器械及其正确使用法,各种缝合方法

【目的和要求】

1. 熟悉常用外科手术器械及其正确使用方法。

2. 学习外科各种缝合方法。

【实习程序】

1. 先认识常用手术器械和手术包,学习外科常用手术器械的使用方法。

2. 外科手术基本器械的正确使用方法和缝合方法,先由教师讲解、示范,然后学生进行适当练习,缝合练习在缝合练习板上进行。

【实习项目】

一、介绍基本外科器械的名称

见图 2-1～图 2-6。

二、外科缝线

1. 理想外科缝线的材质应满足以下条件 ①无菌性;组织反应轻微,不利于细菌生长;②通用性,缝合材料能适用于任何外科手术;③线的作用必须保持到创口愈合为止;④线在伤口愈合后最好能被吸收,同时不引起组织反应;⑤无毛细管作用,无过敏性,无致癌性;⑥打结后能维持组织对合,又无磨损或切割;⑦有足够的摩擦系数,手感好,线结不易松脱;⑧价廉,材质来源充足。然而,这种理想的缝线目前并不存在,所以外科医生必须挑选出一种与这种理想尽可能接近的缝线。

2. 常用外科缝线分类 一般将外科缝线分为:天然和合成,可吸收和不可吸收,以及单股和多股。

(1) 天然与合成:天然材质(如:外科肠线和外科丝线)普遍存在伤口并发症发生率高的缺点,而合成材质缝线所致的组织反应和炎症轻。如今,缝线材料已经逐渐由以前的天然材料向合成材料过渡。

(2) 单股与多股:与多股缝线相比,单股缝线有许多优点:①伤口感染率低。推测其原因是多股缝线的纤维之间存在缝隙,细菌可以藏匿其中,抵御白细胞的吞噬。如果有感染存在,应该选用单股缝线,因为这种缝线没有缝隙,细菌就无从藏匿。金黄色葡萄球菌的直径 $0.7\sim1.2~\mu m$,单核细胞直径 $15\sim20~\mu m$,中性粒细胞直径 $12\sim15~\mu m$。②组织损伤小。单股缝线表面光滑,缝合时对组织无切割作用。③用单股缝线连续缝合腹部切口,每针缝线的受力相等(犹如滑轮组机制),如此,有望减少伤口裂开和切口疝发生。单股缝线的缺

点是容易被器械损伤、手感差、需要多重结以防滑脱。多股（编织）缝线（如丝线、微乔线）在通过组织时会产生**线锯**样切割作用（图 2-14），对组织造成损伤。实验表明，多股缝线造成的炎症反应和胶原酶激活比单股缝线（如 **PDS**、普理灵）重。

（3）可吸收与不可吸收：可吸收缝线的材料有多种，因此，吸收时间各异。长期留在组织内的缝线应选用可吸收线或单股线，不可吸收的编织线对组织有刺激，并且容易藏匿细菌。

（4）合成缝线的规格：一般常用为 000（3-0）、00（2-0）、0、1、2 等几种，缝线型号的确定依据是缝线的直径（表 2-1）。

表 2-1　合成缝线的规格划分

中国规格	USP[1] 规格	EP[2] 规格	最小直径（mm）	最大直径（mm）
	8-0	0.4	0.040	0.049
	7-0	0.5	0.050	0.069
	6-0	0.7	0.070	0.099
3-0	5-0	1.0	0.100	0.149
0	4-0	1.5	0.150	0.199
1	3-0	2.0	0.200	0.249
4	2-0	3.0	0.300	0.339
7	0	3.5	0.350	0.399
10	1	4	0.400	0.499
	2	5	0.500	0.599
	3,4	6	0.600	0.699
	5	7	0.700	0.799

[1] 美国药典（United States Pharmacopoeia，USP），[2] 欧洲药典（European Pharmacopoeia，EP），EP 相当于公制（metric）。

三、外科手术基本器械的正确使用方法

1. **手术刀**　手术刀用来切开和解剖组织，可根据手术部位和性质的不同，更换大小不同的刀片。手术刀由可装卸的刀片和刀柄组成，安装时，左手持刀柄尾端，刀柄的刀片载座向上，用血管钳夹住刀片尖端钝缘，与刀片载座对合后，安装于刀柄上。使用后，用血管钳夹住刀片的尾端，稍提起刀片，向前推开取下（图 2-7）。正确的执刀方式有五种（图 2-8）：

（1）执西餐刀式：为最常用的一种执刀方式，动作范围大而灵活，用于各种胸腹部皮肤切口。用拇指、第三和第四指抓刀身，食指放在刀背上，其动作涉及整个上肢，而力量主要在腕部。

（2）执（琴）弓式：拇指放在刀柄的一侧，其余四指放在刀柄的另一侧。

（3）执笔式：用于切割短小切口，用力轻柔而操作精细便于控制，如解剖血管、神经，切开腹膜小切口等。小刀片往往有助于精细操作。其动作和力量主要在手指。

（4）握持式：刀身抓在手掌中，用于切割范围较广、用力较大的切开，如截肢等。

（5）反挑式：主要用于脓肿切开引流。执笔式握刀，但刀刃向上，将11号刀片刺入脓肿，然后向上挑开，可避免损伤深部组织。

2. 手术剪　分为两大类：一类用于分离、解剖和剪开组织；另一类用于剪断缝线、剪开敷料和引流管等。直剪用于浅表手术，弯剪用于深部手术。正确的执剪姿势如图2-9所示，即将拇指和环指的一部分套入剪刀柄环口中，如此，手臂可以随意做旋前、旋后以及剪切动作。不要将手指伸入剪刀柄的环口太深，妨碍手部做动作。

手术剪在解剖组织时，不外两种作用：一是剪断组织，如剪断已结扎妥善的血管；二是分离，利用剪刀的尖端，插入组织间隙后撑开，分离疏松的粘连和穿通无血管的组织，如系膜、网膜等。

3. 常用外科钳　外科常用的钳有多种，其头部可以是直的，也可以是弯的，半齿或全齿，有齿或无齿（无损伤），以及大、中、小等各种类型。常用来夹闭血管或钳夹组织。最常用的属血管钳。直血管钳用于手术野浅部或皮下止血，弯血管钳用于较深部止血；半齿一般用于腹壁，全齿用于腹腔，蚊式血管钳（最小的一种）用于精细的止血和分离组织。

血管钳主要用于钳夹血管或出血点，以达到止血目的。也用于分离组织、牵引缝线、夹住和拔出缝针等。执血管钳的姿势与执剪刀姿势相同（图2-9）。合拢血管钳时，两手动作相同，但在松开血管钳时，两手操作则不同。右手是用已套入血管钳环口的拇指与无名指相对挤压，继而做旋开的动作开放血管钳。左手则是用拇指与食指捏住血管钳的一个环，中指与无名指顶住另一环，用拇指和无名指稍用力对顶一下，即可开放（图2-10）。血管钳只需夹住血管或出血点即可，避免夹住过多组织。

4. 持针器（钳）　持针钳可以是直的，也可以是弯的。后者主要用于空间受限的深部操作。所需持针钳的大小主要依据针的大小而定。用持针钳的尖端夹持缝针，缝合各种组织。缝针被夹持的部位，应在缝针的中后三分之一交界处，缝针与持针器呈直角（图2-11）。执持针钳的方法有多种，最常用的方法与持剪刀姿势相同（图2-9）。但为了缝合方便，可以抓住柄部和环部，不必将拇指和无名指套入环口中（图2-12）。持针钳可用于打结（图1-16）。

5. 手术镊　主要用于夹住或提起组织，便于剥离、剪开或缝合。手术镊有有齿与无齿之分：前者用于夹较坚韧的组织，如皮肤、筋膜、肌腱等；后者用于夹脆弱的组织，如血管、神经、黏膜等。正确的执镊方法如图2-13，以拇指对食指和中指，适当地用力夹住组织，两手都可以持镊。

6. 拉钩　用于牵拉开手术区表面的组织，充分暴露操作部位，以便进行手术。拉钩可分为手持及自动拉钩两类，根据其用途不同，而有形状及深浅多种型号。在使用拉钩时，必须注意勿用力过猛而损伤组织。对柔软、脆弱的组织，如肝脏以及切口缘，最好在拉钩下方衬以纱布垫。

7. 外科缝针　缝针的作用是引线用于缝合各种组织和贯穿缝扎。根据其缝合组织的不同，缝针有不同的大小和形状。根据其尾部分为有眼针和无眼针，有针眼的缝针穿过组织时造成的损伤大（图2-14，图2-15）。无损伤缝针是将缝线嵌入针尾部。根据弯度不同可分为直针和弯针；弯针根据其弧度不同，又分1/4圆、3/8圆、1/2圆和5/8圆等几种；根据尖端形状的不同，可分为圆针和三角针。三角针有三角形刃缘，锐利，属损伤性缝针，能穿透较坚硬的组织,适用于缝合皮肤及软骨等。圆针细而无刃缘,用于缝合一般软组织,如胃肠道、血管、筋膜、腹膜、神经鞘膜等。

8. **手术器械的传递**　手术器械应该以随即可用的方式递给术者(图 2-16)。当术者拿到器械后马上就能用上,视线不必从手术野移开。手术护士(器械护士)或助手应该明白术者的手势,知道他需要何物。当术者将手伸过来时,能立即把器械放到他手掌的恰当位置,术者收拢手指时恰能抓住器械,并能用上。将手术器械传递给手术人员时,应将刀柄、剪刀把手或血管钳把手递给手术人员。严禁将刀尖或剪刀头部递给手术人员,以免刺伤手术人员。

9. **穿线**(图 2-17)

(1) 用锐剪刀将线头(丝线)剪成 45°,使之容易穿入针眼。

(2) 用水湿润线头,使线头的纤维相互聚拢、挺括,容易穿入针眼。

(3) 左手持针,看清针眼。如针眼不清楚,可在针眼后方放白色物。

(4) 右手的拇指和食指捏住线头垂直穿入针眼,当线头露出针眼后,用右拇指将线头顶在针眼处防止线头退脱;然后,用右食指或左食指压住露出的线头,在右拇指帮助下将线头拖出 8~10 cm。

注意:图是按右利者的手画。左利者可将图对着镜子学习穿线。

四、外科缝合

(一) 常用外科缝合法

缝合的方法很多,但基本的缝合方法有单纯对合缝合、内翻缝合和外翻缝合三类,而每一类中又分为间断缝合和连续缝合二式。重点练习单纯间断缝合、"8"字形缝合、连续缝合和荷包缝合。

1. **单纯间断缝合**(图 2-18)　使组织对合,用于缝合皮肤、皮下组织等。用单纯间断缝合创口时,要使皮缘外翻,避免皮肤张力过大。线结要打在一侧。皮肤的缝合要求将皮缘精准对合。间断缝合与连续缝合的不同点在于间断缝合不会使组织"缩拢"。

2. **双间断缝合**("8"字形缝合)(图 2-19)　使组织对合,用于缝合皮下组织、筋膜、肌腱等组织,有张力缝合作用。

3. **间断垂直褥式缝合**　垂直褥式缝合由一针短边距的浅层缝合和一针长边距的深层缝合组成,它是保证创缘外翻的最佳选择。这种缝合有利于组织外翻,常用于皮肤缝合后容易发生内翻的部位,如:颈项部,肢体凹面的创口以及阴囊皮肤的缝合(图 2-20)。

4. **间断水平褥式缝合**(图 2-21)　主要作用是将伤口拉拢,或对创口起初步固定作用。

5. **单纯连续缝合**(图 2-22)　常用于腹膜缝合。

6. **连续交锁(毯边)缝合**(图 2-23)　常用于胃肠吻合、缝合腹膜或大张游离皮片移植等。

7. **间断浆肌层内翻缝合**(Lembert 缝合)(图 2-24、图 3-6)　常用于胃肠吻合时外层(浆肌层)的缝合。

8. **间断水平褥式浆肌层内翻缝合**(Halsted 缝合)(图 2-25)　用于肠吻合时外层(浆肌

层)缝合。

9. 连续浆肌层内翻缝合(Cushing 缝合)(图 2-26)　这种缝合的方法同 Connell,但是,缝针不穿透黏膜下层和黏膜层。Cushing 缝合用于胃肠吻合时外层(浆肌层)缝合。

10. 连续全层内翻缝合(Connell 缝合)(图 2-27)　用于肠吻合时内层(全层)缝合。

11. 荷包缝合(图 2-28)　用于阑尾残端埋入。

12. 连续水平褥式外翻缝合(图 2-29)　用于缝合血管。

13. Smead-Jones"远—近"缝合(图 2-30)　属张力缝合,常用于腹部缝合。

14. 减张缝合(图 2-31)　在伤口缝合张力较大时应用。

15. 表皮下连续缝合(连续皮内缝合)(图 2-32)　为了消除缝合后所形成的轨道样瘢痕,外科医生可以在真皮上做连续的、短的侧缘缝合。倘若使用的是不吸收缝线,缝线的两端要从切口的两端露出,可以将缝线的两端相互打结形成"环状",也可以各自在两端打结。

(二)组织缝合的基本原则

在无张力状态拉拢切开的组织,消灭空隙,便于伤口愈合。皮肤缝合时应避免边缘内翻。

1. 持针器最好与拟缝合轴线平行(图 2-33)。缝针的力线要与皮肤平面垂直(针尖与皮肤平面呈 80°～100°角)(图 2-34),使缝针容易进入组织,减少缝针断裂的机会。在缝针尖端穿出组织后,建议术者自己用左手(右利者)持手术镊抓取缝针的尖端,尽量不要请助手帮忙夹针。

2. 勿留残腔(死腔)。

3. 正确地组织对合,皮肤缝合时要求皮缘外翻,没有张力(图 2-35)。

4. 切口两侧所包含组织的多少要相等。创缘一侧的进针位置与对侧的出针位置距创缘应等距离(等边距),并且应该位于正对侧。

5. 缝线针数不宜过疏或过密。皮肤缝合时,一般针距为 1 厘米,边距 1 厘米(图 2-36)。

6. 结扎缝线松紧要适当,过松则组织对合不良,过紧则加剧疼痛,引起组织缺血、坏死。

7. 缝合遇到血管出血时,应将缝针退出(尤其当用有眼缝针缝合时),压迫出血处片刻止血,然后重新缝合(图 2-37)。

(三)结扎止血和缝合止血

1. 游离结扎止血

先用血管钳夹住血管断端的两头进行止血。由于血管钳钳夹后的组织有损伤,因此要用血管钳的尖端夹住血管的断端,不要夹带邻近的组织。然后,用线将血管扎住达到止血目的。

将一根线绕过夹住血管的血管钳,打第一个半结(图 1-13-1)。此时,助手应该抓住血管钳,务必使术者能见到血管钳尖端,下压血管钳柄使血管钳尖上翘。在术者第一个半结打紧时,助手松开血管钳,术者继续把第一个半结打紧,然后打第二个半结。

2. 缝合结扎(贯穿结扎,缝扎)

缝扎主要用于重要血管,防止结扎线滑脱。缝扎位置应该距血管断端有足够距离,以防一侧血管壁滑脱出血。常用"8"字缝合法(图 2-38)。如果用无损伤缝线缝针,缝线可以从血管中间穿过，缝线打一道结，扎住血管的一半，然后缝线绕血管一周扎住血管。

（四）剪线

线结打牢后，要剪去过长的线头。剪线过程中要求能看清剪刀尖部，避免无意中剪伤结扎线以外的重要组织。剪线时，线剪头部微张开，剪刀刃沿缝线缓缓下滑至线结处，然后将剪刀顺时针转 45°剪线（右手剪线时）（图 2-39）。

（五）拆线

只有皮肤缝线需要拆线。皮肤缝线应该尽早拆除，前提是组织愈合达到了满意的张力强度。皮肤缝线拆线过晚会在皮肤上遗留难看的轨道样瘢痕。拆线过早又会引起伤口裂开。面部缝线的拆线时间一般是 5 天，手、足和关节部位的缝线一般在 14 天或 14 天后拆除。皮内缝合的缝线晚一些时间拆除也无大碍。拆线时，应注意不使原来显露在皮肤外面的线段经过皮下组织（图 2-40，图 2-41）（拆线操作详见附录五）。

Session 3　Cadaveric jejunal anastomosis（end to end）
　　　　　 & Surgical aseptic techniques（video tape）

【Goals & requirements】

1. Be familiar with methods of suture for gastrointestinal reconstruction: interrupted or continous full-layer inverting suture or Connell suture, and interrupted inverting seromuscular suture or Lembert suture.

2. Review surgical aseptic techniques by watching video tape and cinema.

【Progress schedule】

1. Educator will demonstrate intestinal anastomosis first, and then students will be asked to follow step by step after hand washing, gowning and gloving.

2. Watching video or film.

3. At the end of this session, the educator will present his/her comment.

【Topics of this session】

To enhance suture technique training, two-layer anastomosis are to be used in this session, although interrupted single-layer serosubmucosal suture is the "gold standard" for intestinal anastomosis, which showed faster and sounder healing when compared to the traditional two-layer anastomosis.

In this session, all students will have a segment of cadaveric jejunum which will be cut apart and then reconstructed for practice.

1. A cadaveric jejunal segment to be cut is identified and transected between two Kocher clamps. Two intestinal clamps are placed 3～5 cm away from each Kocher clamp, respectively. The bowel is then divided. The two ends to be anastomosed are placed side by side. The mesenteric and antimesenteric borders of the two segments are apposed respectively.

2. Two seromuscular stay sutures (1/0 silk) were placed through both segments on the mesenteric and antimesenteric borders, respectively, to stabilize the position of the segments relative to each other. Both Kocher clamps are placed parallel each other and turned 90° outward to expose the initial surfaces to be sutured. Make the first posterior interrupted seromuscular suture at the midpoint, 5 mm from the cut edge, through the proximal and distal bowel and tied. The posterior interrupted seromuscular sutures are advanced to the mesenteric edge and then to the antimesenteric edge, or vice versa, at intervals of 5～6 mm (Fig. 3-1).

It is also accepted to make the posterior full-layer suture first, and then the anterior full-layer and anterior outer layer. At last, the anastomosis is turned through 180° to achieve a satisfactory lie. The posterior seromuscular sutures are inserted，working away from the mesenteric edge，thus ending on the anti-mesenteric border.

3. The intestine was transected with a scalpel as close as possible to the Kocher clamp to remove the crushed bowel wall (Fig. 3-2). Then，posterior full-layer sutures are placed using simple interrupted surtures starting with the initial bite as close as possible to mesenteric end and advancing toward the opposite side (Fig. 3-3，Fig. 3-4).

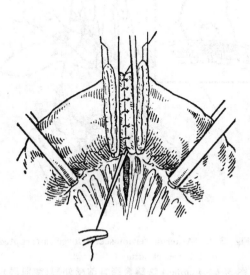

Fig. 3-1   Posterior interrupted seromuscular suture
图 3-1   肠管后壁外层（浆肌层）间断缝合

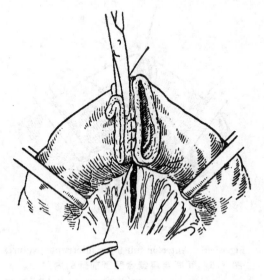

Fig. 3-2   Removing the crushed bowel wall
图 3-2   切去被 Kocher 钳压榨的肠壁

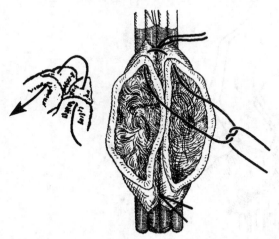

Fig. 3-3   Starting posterior full-layer sutures using simple interrupted surtures
图 3-3   开始肠后壁内层的间断全层缝合

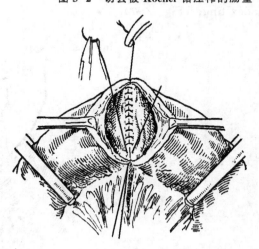

Fig. 3-4   Posterior full-layer interrupted sutures
图 3-4   肠后壁内层的间断全层缝合

4. Once the posterior full-layer of sutures has been completed，stay sutures are tied without cut. Then，anterior full-layer sutures are inserted using simple interrupted surtures starting with the initial bite at the midpoint and advancing toward the both ends

(Fig. 3-5).

    5. Once the anterior full-layer has been closed，the anterior seromuscular layer is sutured with interrupted Lembert sutures （Fig. 3-6）. All remaining sutures are tied and cut，and the mesenteric defect is closed.

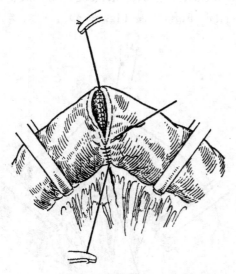

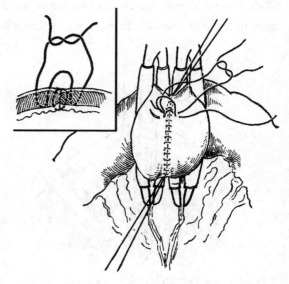

Fig. 3-5　Anterior full-layer interrupted sutures
图 3-5　间断全层缝合肠管前壁的内层

Fig. 3-6　Anterior seromuscular layer interrupted
Lembert sutures
图 3-6　Lembert 法缝合肠管前壁外层（浆肌层）

    6. Check all sutures and knots，and then test patency of the stroma with thumb and index finger(Fig. 3-7).

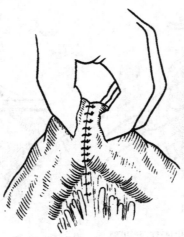

Fig. 3-7　Testing the patency of the stroma with thumb and index finger （pinching-masturbating the anastomosis to confirm an adequate lumen）
图 3-7　拇指和食指试探吻合口通畅情况

    7. The posterior full-layer of suture can be closed with simple continous suture or continous interlocking suture starting with the initial bite as close as possible to the mes-

enteric edge and advancing toward the antimesenteric edge. The same thread is turned to the anterior full-layer of suture using Connell suture from mesenteric edge to antimesenteric edge. Then, the two ends of the thread meet each other and are tied with the knot inside the intestinal lumen (Fig. 3-8, Fig. 3-9).

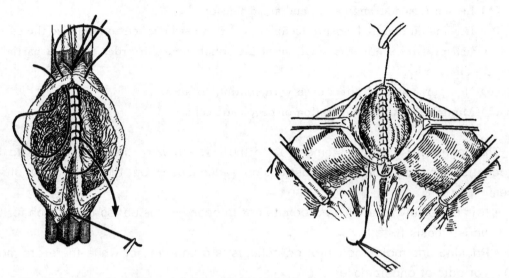

Fig. 3-8   Posterior full-layer continous interlocking suture starting turning to the anterior full-layer Connell suture

图 3-8   肠后壁内层的连续全层毯边缝合,转向前壁的缝法

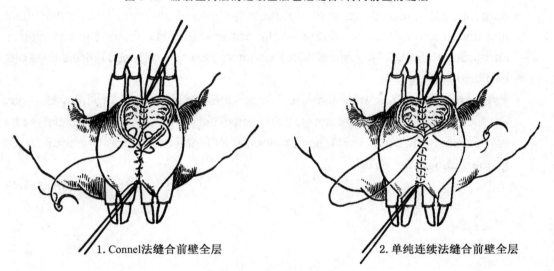

1. Connel法缝合前壁全层   2. 单纯连续法缝合前壁全层

Fig. 3-9   Anterior full-layer continuous suture

1. The same suture is continued interiorly as a Connell suture; 2. The same suture is continued interiorly as a simple running suture.

图 3-9   肠前壁内层的连续全层缝合法

1. 转向前壁后,用同一根线作全层内翻缝合(Connell 法);2. 转向前壁后,用同一根线作全层单纯连续缝合肠管前壁的内层。

8. Tips for intestinal anastomosis：

(1) Accurate tissue apposition.

(2) Incorporate submucosa which is the strongest layer in the gastrointestinal tract.

(3) Minimize damage to sub mucosal vascular plexus.

(4) Lessen tissue strangulation and avoid tension.

(5) If using an inverted closure technique, care must be taken to minimize the cuff of tissue which protrudes into the small sized intestinal lumen in order to avoid partial or complete obstruction.

(6) No 'purse string' effect even with continuous suture.

(7) Minimize risk of implantation of neoplastic cells.

The gastrointestinal anastomosis is to the surgeon what the parachute is to the parachutist. Both can fail with disastrous consequences — but there are a few differences.

- It is extremely rare for a parachute not to open — it is not so uncommon for the anastomosis to fail.
- Packing and maintenance of parachutes is a uniform act while there are many variants of anastomoses.
- Opening a parachute is a simple, standardized undertaking — fashioning an anastomosis is a little more complex.
- Surgeons often lose sleep worrying about the fate of the anastomosis they have just constructed (I do!). But when the parachute fails no one is left to worry. Fortunately, for us, surgeons, when anastomoses fail somebody else's lives are in mortal danger.
- When the parachutist dies there is no one to remember but his family, but the surgeon will remember the anastomotic leak and its consequences — unless he is a psychopath. And if he doesn't manage the leak satisfactorily he may be reminded about it in court!

Moshe Schein

实习三 离体猪肠端对端吻合术、外科无菌技术和基本操作复习(放教学电影和电视录像)

【目的和要求】

1. 熟悉胃肠道缝合的几种主要方法:间断或连续全层内翻缝合(Connell 缝合)、间断浆肌层内翻缝合(Lembert 缝合)。

2. 通过放教学电影和电视录像,较全面、系统地复习外科无菌技术和手术基本操作,为以后的动物手术实习做好准备。

【实习程序】

1. 教师示教后,学生按照无菌手术程序和要求,进行手术人员的术前准备和手术区(教具)的准备,然后进行离体猪肠端对端吻合的练习,每人进行一次肠吻合术。

2. 观看教学电影和电视录像。

3. 肠吻合术教学结束后,由教师点评、小结。

【实习项目】

尽管一层间断浆膜—黏膜下缝合与既往的两层缝合相比愈合快、质量好,已经被看做胃肠吻合的"金标准"。但是,为了增加学生动手操作锻炼的机会,本次离体肠吻合实习仍然练习两层吻合。

本次实习中,每位学生会得到一段离体肠管,并进行切断和吻合重建练习。

1. 取猪肠一段,紧贴拟切断线两侧各夹一把 Kocher 钳,再在 Kocher 钳外侧距 Kocher 钳 3~5 cm 处分别用肠钳一把夹住后离断肠管,助手将两断端靠拢,肠系膜缘对肠系膜缘。

2. 先在两段肠壁的肠系膜缘和对肠系膜缘,用 1 号丝线穿过浆肌层各缝一针,作为牵引固定。两把 Kocher 钳并排放置、向外旋转 90°,暴露肠后壁拟缝合区。在肠后壁的中点处开始,作第一针间断浆肌层缝合,距离切缘(边距)约 0.5 cm。然后向两端做缝合,每针间距(针距)约 0.5 cm(图 3-1)。

肠后壁的浆肌层缝合,也可待后壁全层、前壁全层和前壁浆肌层缝合完毕后,再将后壁翻转向前最后进行。

3. 接着切去被 Kocher 钳压榨的肠壁(图 3-2),作肠后壁的间断全层缝合,每针间距同前(图 3-3,图 3-4)。

4. 后壁全层缝合完毕,牵引线打结,仍作牵引用。从中间开始,以同样的间断全层缝合方法向两端缝合前壁的内层(图 3-5)。

5. 待前壁全层缝合完毕,放开肠钳,最后用 Lembert 法缝合前壁浆肌层(图 3-6)。所有缝线打结,剪去线头,缝闭系膜孔。

6. 检查前、后壁缝合处是否均匀可靠。以拇指和食指试探吻合口的大小(图 3-7)。

7. 肠后壁全层亦可从对肠系膜缘开始,用肠线作全层连续缝合或毯边缝合,至肠系膜缘时再转向前壁,用同一根线作全层内翻缝合(Connell 缝合),缝至对肠系膜缘,与起始处的缝线会合,最后线结打在肠腔内(图 3-8,图 3-9)。

8. 肠吻合要点

(1) 正确对合。

(2) 黏膜下层是胃肠道诸层中最坚韧的一层,胃肠吻合时一定要缝合该层。

(3) 尽可能减少对黏膜下血管丛的损伤。

(4) 减少组织缺血,避免吻合口张力。

(5) 内翻缝合时,组织不能翻入肠腔过多,以免发生肠梗阻。

(6) 连续缝合时要避免"收拢"效应。

(7) 防止肿瘤细胞种植。

胃肠吻合与外科医生的关系就好比降落伞与跳伞员的关系。两者都可能因为失败出现灾难性后果,两者的不同点如下:

- 降落伞打不开的概率极低,而吻合失败并不少见。

- 降落伞的打包和维护程序是千篇一律的,而吻合的变数极大。

- 打开降落伞的程式是简单的、标准化的,而吻合则有点复杂。

- 外科医生往往会因为对刚结束的吻合顾虑重重、彻夜难眠(我就是这样!)。而如果降落伞未能打开,则不会有人提心吊胆。就我们外科医生来讲这是幸运,因为,在生死线上挣扎的是他人。

- 跳伞员死后除了他的家人,没有人会怀念他;而外科医生会记得每个吻合口漏及其结局,除非他是一个心理变态的外科医生。但是,如果他在吻合口漏上出了纰漏,法庭会让他回忆这件事!

Moshe Schein

Session 4　First-aid for trauma

【Goals & requirements】

1. To be familiar with the START triage system and the correct use of START tag. Know the important role of cervical spine protection in the first aid to a victim with blunt trauma.

2. To be familiar with the three most commonly used techniques of bandaging — spiral technique, figure-of-eight technique and spiral reversed bandage technique.

3. Know the proper procedures to assist an external bleeding victim

【Progress schedule】

1. Students are divided into two groups. The students assigned to Block A will learn bandaging techniques and the students in Block B START triage system, cervical spine protection and bleeding control by watching video or film. After 2 hours, the two groups exchange their tasks each other.

2. Educator will demonstrate the techniques first, and then students will be asked to follow step by step.

3. At the end, educator will present his/her comment.

【Topics of this session】

A.　Simple Triage and Rapid Transport (START)

1. START Triage　Assessment of the trauma patient should follow an orderly script, addressing first the life-threatening problems: **A**irway, **B**reathing, **C**irculation, and neurologic **D**isability (see Session 5). Failure to follow the ABCD of the primary survey for the multiply injured patient may seriously jeopardize survival; initial attention should not be directed toward the most dramatically obvious injury such as a mangled extremity.

Please note, START Triage is an initial assessment tool during a mass casualty incident (MCI) and should not be used for extended patient holding areas (trauma center or hospital). Once patients are received into treatment and holding areas, a more thorough assessment and triage process should be performed. **Remember, during an MCI, it is critical to rapidly identify all injured patients and categorize them appropriately. This is the best way to ensure that everyone receives the care they need during the MCI.**

START identifies those patients that will die within the first hour. This includes patients with injuries such as respiratory compromise, shock and altered mental status. Since

START triage does not have to be performed by the highest level provider, thus freeing this provider to be utilized in the treatment area. First, start with scene size up, before you get into the "thick of things" radio your dispatch center.

START Triage is based on three assessment criteria (respiration, pulse and mental status), which will lead you into placing the patient in one of four triage categories:

□ **Minor（Green）**: These patients are the walking wounded and need to be seen at a hospital or prompt care clinic within twelve to twenty-four hours. Evacuation of these casualties is not usually a priority. In addition, these patients may be used in assisting EMS providers in patient care.

□ **Delayed（Yellow）**: These patients cannot walk due to mental or traumatic injuries. These patients need to be evacuated to a hospital within two hours.

□ **Immediate（Red）**: These patients need being transported as soon as possible. These casualties have life-threatening injuries that must be cared for within one hour.

□ **Deceased（Black）**: These patients are clinically dead with no pulse and no respirations. This includes patients with obvious mortal injuries such as head injuries with exposed brain matter.

The START Triage System

1st step	Direct all patients within the sound of your voice to walk out of the incident area and towards you[1]. These patients are considered to be in the **Minor** category (**Green**), and everyone who can not walk to you will either be **Delayed**（YELLOW）, **Immediate**（RED） or **Deceased**（BLACK）
2nd step	assess respiration of the remaining victims who can not walk to you[2] ● no respiratory effect after opening airway　　　　**Deceased**（BLACK） ● respirations＞30　　　　**Immediate**（RED） ● respirations＜30　　　　**Delayed**（YELLOW）
3rd step	assess tissue perfusion[3] ● no radial pulse present　　　　**Immediate**（RED） ● radial pulse present　　　　**Delayed**（YELLOW）
4th step	assess neurological statues ● unconscious　　　　**Immediate**（RED） ● cannot follow simple commands[4]　　　　**Immediate**（RED） ● can follow simple commands　　　　**Delayed**（YELLOW）

Notes:

1. Research shows those who can "walk and talk" after a MCI are probably not critically injured.

2. Start where you stand and assess the patients one by one. Do not go towards patients that look critically injured and thus stepping over those who do not appear injured. Zigzagging triage patterns will increase the chance of missing patients. You should only stop triage to open an airway or stop a killer bleed. Any further treatment will delay triage and could result in the mass of patients not receiving care in a timely manner. As you move through the scene, affix a triage tag to each patient according to their priority (Fig. 4-1).

3. Perfusion checks can be completed by skin color and temperature, capillary refill or pulse check at the radial (a non-perfusing radial pulse would present as no pulse or pulse rate greater than 120 / min).

4. Simple commands, like "touch your nose", "can you take a deep breath?", or simple questions, like "what happened?", "where it hurts the most?".

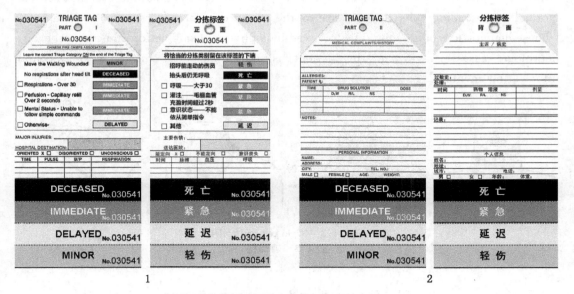

1   2

Fig. 4-1　START Triage tag
1. front; 2. back
图 4-1　START 分拣标签
1. 正面;2. 反面

2. Recovery position (Fig. 4-2)　Keep the victim lying flat, with the head at the level of the body. Do not raise the feet if the face is flushed. If the victim is having trouble breathing, you may raise the head slightly. Watch closely for vomiting and position the head to avoid getting vomit or saliva into the lungs.

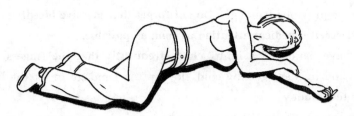

Fig. 4-2　Recovery position
图 4-2　休息体位

B. Cervical spine protection

Blunt trauma patients, especially the patients with pain on the posterior neck, should be assumed to have sustained a cervical spine injury until proven otherwise by an unequivocal physical examination and radiographic survey. Spinal immobilization with **a rigid cer-**

vical collar（Fig. 4-3）and a long spine board should be performed immediately in these patients until their mental status has improved and a normal examination is demonstrated. Normal spine radiographs do not ensure the absence of transverse ligament rupture. （These diagnostic studies should be followed by a physical examination and comprehensive neurologic assessment when the patient is not under the influence of alcohol/intoxicating agents.）

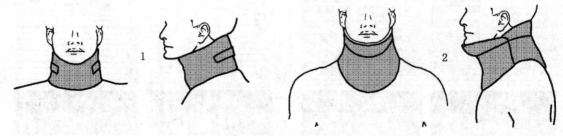

Fig. 4-3 Rigid cervical collar
图 4-3 硬颈托

C. Basic bandage techniques

（A）First aid in external bleeding

1. The principles：

（1）**Press hard onto the wound** to stop the bleeding.

（2）If an arm or leg is cut，**elevate the limb.**

（3）**Cover with a clean pad** and apply a bandage.

（4）Check that the bleeding has stopped. If it has not，add another pad，and bandage，do not remove previous bandage. **Do not forget that massive bleeding，and any deep or large wound must receive medical attention as soon as possible.**

（5）If you have bandaged a limb，**check frequently that the fingers and toes remain warm.** If fingers and toes are getting cold，loosen the bandage to let the blood circulate.

2. Pressing techniques

（1）Directly pressing onto the wound is the usual way to control bleeding，either with the hand directly or with a dressing of some sort（bandage，handkerchief etc.）.

（2）Special pressure points：It is sometimes not possible to press directly on a wound. For example，there may be a foreign body inside the wound，or a broken bone protruding outside，or the wound may be too large or be inaccessible（e. g. if the limb is trapped by some immovable object）. In this case，the only way to control the bleeding is to compress blood vessels over particular pressure points（usually where arteries cross over bones near to the surface of the skin）. This technique can be used to control external bleeding from the wounds of head，face，arm or leg（Fig. 4-4 to Fig. 4-6）.

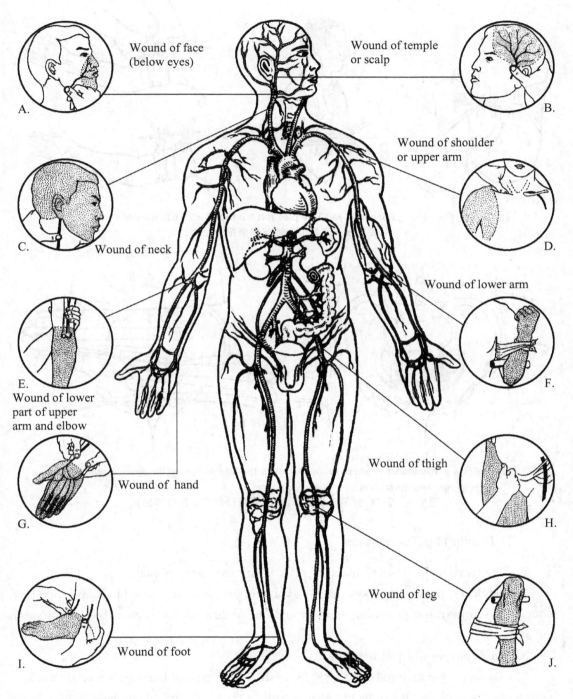

Wound of face (below eyes)

Wound of temple or scalp

Wound of shoulder or upper arm

A.

B.

Wound of neck

C.

D.

Wound of lower arm

E.

F.

Wound of lower part of upper arm and elbow

Wound of hand

Wound of thigh

G.

H.

Wound of foot

Wound of leg

I.

J.

Fig. 4-4   Special pressure points

图 4-4   特定压迫止血点

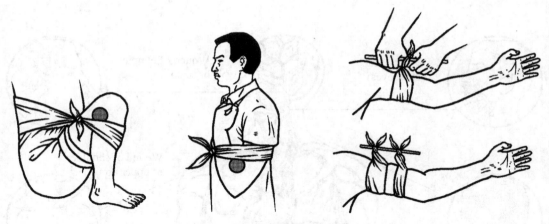

Fig. 4-5　Triangular bandage plus roll bandage for bleeding control
图 4-5　三角巾加纱布绷带用于止血

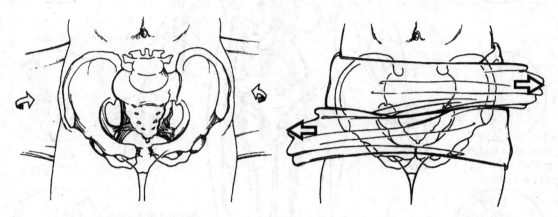

Fig. 4-6　A pelvic binder or sheet wrapped around the hips to reduce the space available for hematoma formation
图 4-6　骨盆兜(用床单制作)用于控制骨盆骨折移位和出血

(B) Bandaging Techniques

1. The three main types of bandage roll, triangular, and tubular.

2. Bandages have three key uses: applying pressure to stop bleeding; covering wounds and burns; and providing support and immobilization for broken bones, sprains, and strains.

3. Material types of roll bandage

(1) Gauze: This material, in a 32×28 mesh, is the type of bandage generally used to hold dressings in place. It can be obtained in rolls 4.8, 6, 8, and 10 cm wide. There is also a variety of "special" bandaging materials. In the main, these are made in such a manner that they "give" in different directions, so as to allow firm application of the bandage even if the proper principles of bandaging have not been observed. These special materials are

more expensive than ordinary gauze and in the hands of an expert they do not produce a better dressing. However, they do make up for the shortcomings of an inexperienced bandager.

(2) Muslin: Muslin may be obtained in 7.5, 10 and 12.5 cm widths. This is used as straps (as the T-binders of the perineum) and to hold traction tape in place on extremities. The advantages of muslin roll are strong, washable and reusable. It can be used for stabilizing extremities, or holding dressings or splints in place.

"T" Bandage: A firm material, such as muslin, is used to hold perineal and scrotal dressings in place. Secure the horizontal limb of the T about the abdomen at the waist with the vertical limb in the midline posteriorly. Cover the wound with gauze squares. Hold these in place with the vertical limb of the T which is brought anteriorly between the legs and tied to the horizontal limb at the waist. For male patients the the vertical limb is bifurcated and one portion is brought up on either side of the scrotum.

(3) Cotton Elastic Bandage: A cotton bandage, so woven that it has considerable elastic properties, has become very popular. It is available in 5, 7.5, 10 and 12.5 cm widths. It can be rapidly, snugly and neatly applied regardless of previous experience; the elastic properties of the dressing allow it to conform to the contour of any portion of the body being dressed. It is used to give support and to apply even pressure. These bandages are expensive, but they can be washed, dried, and reused.

(4) Elastic Adhesive Bandage: This type has considerable value for fixation of dressings in areas where it is difficult to hold a bandage in place and where expansion and contraction are necessary. e. g. , the chest. This type of bandage has a tendency to unroll at the end, a deficiency the bandager can overcome by placing a piece of plain adhesive plaster over each end or by rounding the ends of the elastic adhesive bandage.

4. Methods of roll bandaging　There are various bandaging techniques, each specifically targeting a particular area of the body or a particular type of ailment.

(1) Circular Bandage: This is used over a tubular area, usually about the wounds at the limbs, and forehead or occiput. The bandage is fixed by several turns about the part (Fig. 4-7, Fig. 4-8).

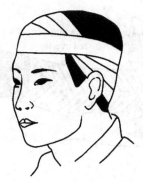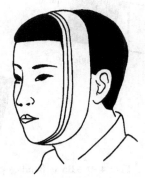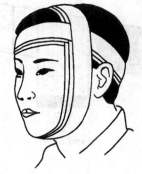

Fig. 4-7　Circular bandage for head
图 4-7　头部环形绷扎法

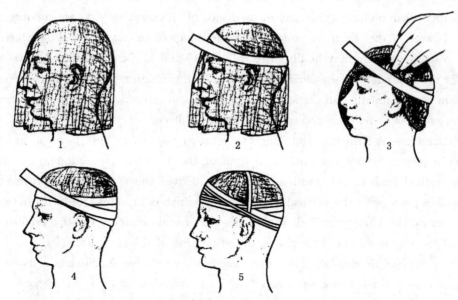

Fig. 4-8　Circular bandage for extensive wounds of the scalp

1. For more extensive wounds of the scalp, a piece of gauze approximately 50 cm square is draped over the head. 2. This is anchored at the level of the forehead by two turns of 5 cm roller bandage. 3. The gauze is turned up over the bandage toward the top of the head. 4. Several more turns of gauze secure this and the dressing is completed by application of adhesive strips.

图 4-8　环形绷扎法（头皮广泛损伤）

1. 头皮的广泛损伤，可以用一块约 50 cm 见方的纱布盖在头部；2. 然后用 5 cm 宽的绷带卷在前额水平固定纱布块；3. 将纱布块的下边反折至绷带的上方至头顶；4. 再继续用绷带缠绕几圈固定纱布块，用胶布固定绷带尾端。

（2）Spiral Bandage：Spiral bandaging is the simplest of the roller bandaging techniques and most often used on body parts with uniform circumference, such as fingers, upper arm or low part of leg. The bandage is fixed by several turns about the part and it is then advanced by circular turns in the direction desired. Each successive turn overlaps the preceding one by 1/3 to 1/2 width. If it begins to be loose at one edge; the bandage may be tightened by applying a reverse spiral (the bandage is rotated clockwise 180 degrees) (Fig. 4-9-1).

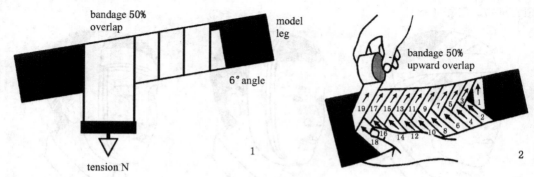

Fig. 4-9　Basic bandages

1. spiral bandage; 2. spiral reversed bandage

图 4-9　基本绷带包扎技术

1. 螺旋绷扎法；2. 螺旋反折绷扎法

（3）Spiral Reversed Bandage：This bandage is most often used on body parts with varying circumference, such as forearm, leg or thigh. The bandage is fixed by two or three circular turns and then, on each turn, a spiral bandage is applied with a reverse turn in order to fit more snugly the varying contours and dimensions of a limb, creating a reverse spiral as it is advanced along the extremity (Fig. 4-9-2, Fig. 4-10-8). **This bandage is likely to slip and is unsuitable for use over joints.**

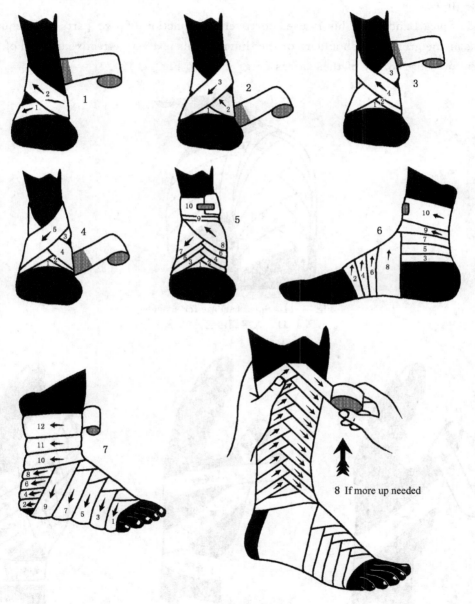

Fig. 4-10 Basic bandages

1～6. figure-of-eight bandage；7. spiral bandage；8. spiral reversed bandage

图 4-10 基本绷带包扎技术

1～6. "8"字绷扎法；7. 螺旋绷扎法；8. 螺旋反折绷扎法

（4）Figure-of-eight Bandage：**Used over joints**，it is anchored at one end by making several turns about the limb below the joint. The bandage is then carried obliquely across the joint and is again anchored above the joint by a complete turn. The dressing is then taken obliquely across the joint to the lower part of the extremity and again anchored with a complete turn. This process is repeated until coverage is adequate. A joint should never be covered by a circular turn unless an elastic bandage is used. （Fig. 4－10－1 to Fig. 4－10－6）

（5）Spica Bandage：This is used to cover the junction of two parts of unequal size such as at the groin，the shoulder，or the thumb. This is a very effective method of applying firm pressure to any of these areas （Fig. 4－11 to Fig. 4－13）.

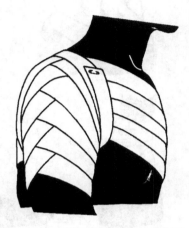

Fig. 4-11　Spica bandage for shoulder
图 4-11　人字绷带包扎（肩部）

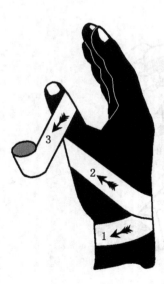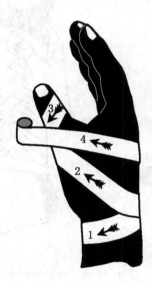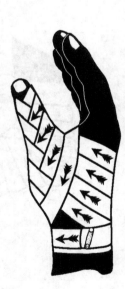

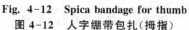

Fig. 4-12　Spica bandage for thumb
图 4-12　人字绷带包扎（拇指）

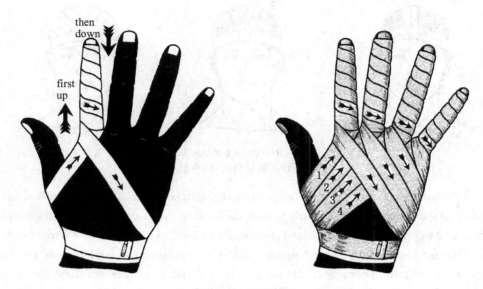

Fig. 4-13   Spiral bangdage plus spica bandage for finger
图 4-13   螺旋绷扎法加人字绷带包扎法（手指）

（6）Recurrent Bandage：This bandage is used on a distal stump, such as finger, toe, head, or amputation stump, that is turned lengthwise to cover the end of the stump and is secured in place by circular turn (Fig. 4-14 to Fig. 4-15).

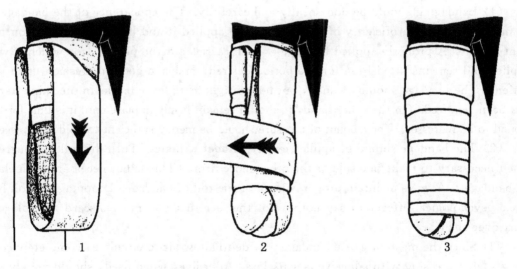

Fig. 4-14   Recurrent bandage for a distal stump
图 4-14   回返绷扎法（截肢残端）

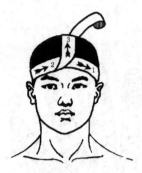 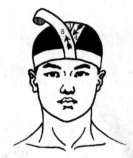 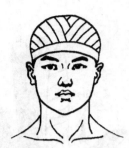

Fig. 4-15　Recurrent bandage for head
图 4-15　回返绷扎法（头部）

5. Triangular bandages　These are amongst the most versatile of all items of first aid equipment. Usually made of washable cotton cloth, they are also available in a disposable paper form. In its open form, a triangular bandage can be used as a sling or as a cover bandage.

6. Tubular bandages　These bandages come in several sizes. Larger ones are used to support joints or hold dressings in place, smaller tubular bandages are ideal for finger or toe injuries. It comes with its own applicator and is best secured with tape.

（1）Cut two and half times the length of the finger or toe to be bandaged and push all of this on to the applicator.

（2）Place the dressing over the wound. Slide the applicator over the finger or toe.

（3）Hold the gauze at the base of the finger or toe and pull the applicator upward, covering the finger or toe with one layer of gauze.

7. General Considerations of Bandaging

（1）Bandaging should be done neatly and carefully. The appearance of the bandage is an indication of the proficiency of the person who applied it and has an effect also on patient morale. A properly applied bandage, which carries out the purpose for which it was applied and remains in position for the period desired, makes a good impression upon the patient. The bandage should be snug, but not so tight as to leave marks in the skin after it has been removed. On the other hand, it should remain firmly in place until it is time for the wound to be redressed. The amount of pressure should be merely sufficient to hold it in place.

（2）The bandage should be applied evenly **without wrinkles.** Turn the roll 180 degrees when necessary to make one side or the other more firm. (This is not necessary with elastic bandage.) Always maintain proper control of the roll of bandage. Dropping the roll has a bad psychological effect, to say nothing of the fact that you must discard the roll and start over again.

（3）Since the mesh of gauze bandage is wide to allow air to circulate, completely covering such a dressing with adhesive is senseless. Adhesive, when used, should merely secure the end of the bandage to help hold it in place. When applied over a gauze bandage on an extremity **the adhesive is best wrapped in a spiral** to avoid constriction of the circulation. There is a common tendency to use bandage that is too narrow. Use the widest bandage with which you can properly do the job; for example, 2.5 cm bandage should only be used in wrapping the fingers; 5 cm bandage should be used on the hand and in head dressings. For all other areas, 7. 5 cm bandages should be used with the exception, of course, of the feet where 2. 5 and 5 cm widths are indicated on the toes and foot.

(4) An elastic bandage should not be stretched to its limit before it is applied, or it becomes, in essence, a nonelastic bandage. When used to wrap an extremity, the elastic bandage should be tightest at the distal end and looser as it is applied proximally. It should never be so tight as to leave marks when it is removed. An elastic bandage on the lower extremity must extend to the toes; otherwise the unbandaged limb distal to the elastic dressing will swell. If pressure over a wound is required, additional dressings should be applied and the bandage wrapped tighter. However, under such circumstances the area must be examined at frequent intervals to ensure that the pressure is not injuring the tissues.

(5) Check circulation: Bandages can cut off circulation, particularly as the injury swells. When bandaging, leave an area of skin exposed below the site (fingers or toes) of the injury to enable regular checks of circulation. Check circulation below the site of the bandaging immediately after treatment and every 10 minutes thereafter. Look and feel for the signs and symptoms of reduced circulation. Gently squeeze the skin or the nail bed below the site injury and bandaging until the color disappears from the skin. When pressure is released, the color should return swiftly (color returns as the small blood vessels, the capillaries, refill with blood). If color does not return quickly, circulation may be restricted.

If there are signs that circulation is restricted, gently loosen the bandage (s). If the bandage is covering a wound or burn, do not remove dressings. If it is supporting a broken bone, take care to support the injury as you loosen and re-tie the bandage.

(6) In extremities, bandage is wrapped from distal to proximal except the hand and maintaining joints in a position of function is appreciated (Fig. 4-16).

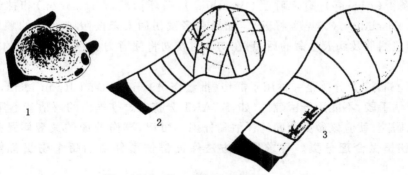

Fig. 4-16　Recurrent bandage for hand

1. To apply a pressure dressing to the hand, first cover the wound, then put gauze between the fingers and place a large amount of mechanic's waste over the palm of the hand and about the fingers. 2. Put the hand in a position of function and cover the entire hand and the wrist with several layers of loose gauze dressing, which is circular over the wrist and recurrent over the hand. 3. Cover the entire dressing with a 5~7 cm cotton elastic bandage. The dressing should be put on in a manner that will allow you to get at the tips of the fingers to ascertain that the circulation is not compromised.

图 4-16　回返绷扎法(手部加压包扎)

1. 先用敷料覆盖伤口,然后用纱布将手指隔开,在手心和手指处放大量碎纱布;2. 将手置于功能位,再用纱布绷带在手和腕部松松地绕几圈;3. 再用弹力绷带包扎。最好能将手指爪节外露,以便观察血供。

实习四　创伤病人的基本急救技术

【目的和要求】

1. 熟悉 START 分拣方法和钝性外伤病人颈椎保护。

2. 熟悉三种最常用的纱布绷带卷包扎法：螺旋绷扎法、螺旋反折绷扎法和"8"字绷扎法。

3. 学习外出血常用的止血方法。

【实习程序】

1. 同学分两组。一组同学学习纱布绷带的应用和包扎方法后，同学之间两两相互练习三种常用的包扎方法，要求动作正确、熟练。另一组同学通过看录像或电影学习 START 分拣方法和硬颈托的使用，以及外科病人的止血和转运。2 小时后两组同学交换学习任务。

2. 教师先做示教，然后，要求学生一步一步跟着学做，直至熟练。

3. 最后，教师做点评。

【实习项目】

一、简单分拣和快速运送（START）

1. **START 分拣系统**　创伤病人的评估应该遵循一定的规律，先找出是否存在致命问题：气道通畅否（Airway）、有无呼吸（Breathing）、循环情况（Circulation）和神经损伤情况（neurologic Disability）（详见实习五）。如果在多发伤病人未按照 ABCD 的顺序进行初次筛查就可能遗漏危及病人生命的后患；在初诊时切勿将注意力放在夺人眼球的损伤上，如：离断的残肢。

请注意：START 分拣是一种用于群伤（批量伤员）（mass casualty incident，MCI）情况下的初始评估手段，不能用于医院内（如：START 分拣对颈椎损伤的评估就不深入）。伤员一旦被送入医院，就应该做更全面的评估和分拣。**切记，群伤处理的关键问题是尽快找出伤员，并对伤员做合理分类。寻求最佳方法保证群伤事件中的每个伤员都能得到恰当救治。**

START 的目标是找出 1 小时内可能发生死亡的伤员，包括呼吸异常、休克以及意识有改变的伤员。START 不要求高水平的专业人员参与，可以让高水平的专业人员腾出手来在治疗区域进行专业处置。首先，是了解事故现场范围，与有关部门取得联系。

START 分拣是基于**三项评估技巧：呼吸、脉搏和意识状态**。根据这三项标准，你可以把伤员分成四类：

□ **轻伤（绿色）**：是能走动的伤员，需要在 12～24 小时内到医院或临时救治诊所进行处理，一般不需要优先运送。这些病人也适合于在医疗急救体系提供的救护站进行处理。

　　□ **延迟救治**（黄色）：是指因意识或受伤而不能行走的伤员。这些伤员需要在 2 小时内送至医院。

　　□ **立即救治**（红色）：是一些需要尽快送至医院的伤员。这些伤员有危及生命的损伤，必须在 1 小时内得到处理。

　　□ **死人**（黑色）：是指没有脉搏和呼吸的临床死亡伤员，包括有显著致命伤的伤员，如头颅外伤伴脑组织外露。

START 分拣系统

第 1 步	在现场喊话，请能走动的伤员走过来。这些伤员归类为**轻伤**（绿色）[1]，其余不能走过来的伤员不是**延迟救治**（黄色），就是**立即救治**（红色），此外就是**死人**（黑色）	
第 2 步	对其他伤员进行呼吸评估[2]	
	● 在开放呼吸道后仍然没有呼吸	**死人**（黑色）
	● 呼吸＞30	**立即救治**（红色）
	● 呼吸＜30	**延迟救治**（黄色）
第 3 步	组织灌注评估[3]	
	● 桡动脉搏动消失	**立即救治**（红色）
	● 桡动脉搏动存在	**延迟救治**（黄色）
第 4 步	神经系统评估	
	● 意识消失	**立即救治**（红色）
	● 不能按简单指令做动作[4]	**立即救治**（红色）
	● 能按简单指令做动作	**延迟救治**（黄色）

注：

1. 这一点（让伤员走动）与协议（规范）可能有抵触，但是，研究表明在 MCI 中，若伤员能"走动和交谈"一般都不会有危及生命的损伤。

2. 从你的立足处开始对伤员逐一进行分拣。不要走向那些看似危重的伤员而忽略那些貌似没有伤的伤员。不要走锯齿形的分拣路线，以免遗漏伤员。仅当需要开放气道或控制致命性大出血时分拣人员才能暂停分拣工作。因为任何进一步的处理都会耽搁分拣工作，导致大批伤员错失抢救良机。每个病人在分拣过后，都戴上相应的颜色标签（图 4-1）。

3. 灌注的评估手段有多种，如：皮肤的色泽和皮温、毛细血管充盈时间或桡动脉搏动（桡动脉触不到搏动提示没有脉搏或脉率大于 120/分钟）。

4. 简单的指令（如："摸一下你的鼻子"，"深吸一口气"），或回答一个简单问题（如："怎么受伤的"，"哪里最痛"）。

　　2. 休息体位（图 4-2）　将伤者平卧，头部与身体处于同一水平。如果面部有血色，就不必抬高下肢。如果伤者有呼吸困难，可以将头部稍抬高。密切注视伤者是否有呕吐，将头部偏向一侧以免吐出物或唾液进入肺内。

二、颈椎保护

　　对钝性伤伤员（尤其是那些外伤后有颈项部疼痛的病人）都应该考虑颈椎损伤的可能，除非体格检查和 X 线检查排除了这种可能性。应该**立即给这些病人戴硬颈托**（图 4-3）**和躺在长硬板床上**，直至意识状态恢复，且体格检查正常。脊柱 X 线检查正常并不能排除环椎横韧带破裂。摄片要与体格检查和神经系统检查一并分析，前提是病人神志清楚，没有酒精或药物中毒。

三、基本绷带包扎技术

（一）外出血的紧急处理

1. 原则

（1）**用力压迫出血处**以达到压迫止血目的。

（2）四肢外伤出血时，可以**抬高伤肢**。

（3）在伤口上**盖清洁敷料**，用绷带包扎。

（4）看看出血是否已经停止。如果依旧有血液从敷料上渗出，追加盖敷料加压包扎，不要移去原有敷料。**将大出血病人迅速转至创伤外科中心处理**。

（5）在四肢用绷带包扎后，要**不时检查手指或足趾的温度**。如果手指或足趾变冷，应该松开绷带，改善伤肢血供。

2. 压迫止血技术

（1）直接压迫：一般的方法是直接在创口上压迫止血，可以用手直接压迫，也可以借助敷料（如：绷带或手帕）。

（2）特殊止血点：有些伤口根本无法使用直接压迫法止血，如：伤口内存在异物、伤口内有骨端外露、伤口太大无法压迫或肢体被卡在某种器物中。此时，止血的唯一方法是压迫特定的止血点（通常是位于皮下的、行走于骨表面的动脉）。这种技术常用于四肢和头面部的伤口出血（图 4-4～图 4-6）。

（二）绷带技术

1. 绷带的主要种类　卷轴绷带（卷带）、三角巾和套筒形绷带。

2. 绷带的主要用途　压迫止血、固定覆盖伤口的敷料和固定伤肢。

3. 卷轴绷带材质种类

（1）纱布绷带：其网眼目数是 32×28，常用于固定伤口敷料。纱布绷带卷的宽度规格有 4.8 cm、6 cm、8 cm 和 10 cm 几种。此外，还有一些"特殊"材料的绷带，制成不同的形状用于不同部位。对绷带"高手"来讲，这些特殊绷带除了价格昂贵外，并无任何优势。但是，对于一位绷带技术不过硬的人来讲，这些特殊绷带确实能弥补他们的不足。

（2）薄棉布绷带：薄棉布绷带的宽度有 7.5 cm、10 cm 和 12.5 cm 几种。薄棉布还可以制作成条状的布带（如用于会阴部的丁字带、腹带、胸带），也可以用于四肢牵引带的固定棉布卷带质料坚固，可用于加压止血或固定肢体、敷料及夹板等。薄棉布绷带耐洗，可反复使用，较为经济。

丁字带：由双层薄棉布制成，用于固定会阴部的敷料或悬吊阴囊。使用时将丁字带的竖带放在腰部后方的中央，将横带在腰部系紧。伤口处盖上方纱布后，将竖带经两腿之间绕至前方，系于丁字带横带的腹侧部。丁字带分男用和女用两种。男用丁字带竖带的下半部是分叉的，可以绕过阴囊和阴茎。

（3）棉质弹力绷带：这是一种棉质绷带，特殊的针织赋予其弹性，因此，颇受外科医生青睐。棉质弹力绷带的宽度有 5 cm、7.5 cm、10 cm 和 12.5 cm 几种。这种绷带的优点是几乎不需要培训就能运用自如、得心应手,适用于身体的任何部位,既可以用于支持,也可以用于压迫。这种绷带的价格贵一些,但是可以洗涤、晾干后重复使用。

(4)弹性自粘绷带:这种绷带的最大优点是可以用于其他绷带不容易固定(容易滑动、移位)的部位,以及需要不时伸缩的部位,如胸部。这种绷带的缺点是尾端容易翘起,因此需要用一小块普通胶布粘贴、固定其尾端。

4. 绷带卷包扎法　绷带卷包扎有许多不同的方法,每种方法都有其特定的使用部位或特定情况。

(1)环形绷扎法:用于肢体较短或圆柱形的部位,如臂部、额部和枕部。环形绷扎法就是在这些部位扎几圈(图4-7,图4-8)。

(2)螺旋绷扎法:螺旋绷扎法是绷带卷包扎术中最简单的方法。主要用于肢体周径均等之部位,如手指、上臂和小腿下段,卷带斜旋上行或下行,每周盖过前周1/3或1/2(图4-9-1)。如果在包扎过程中发现绷带的一侧松开,提示肢体的粗细差异大,需要采用螺旋反折绷扎法。

(3)螺旋反折绷扎法:这种包扎法用于周径差异悬殊的圆形部位,如前臂、小腿和大腿。开始时先做两周环形绷扎,再做螺旋绷扎,然后以一手拇指按住卷带上方正中处,另一手将卷带自该点反折向下,盖过前面1/3或1/2,每次反折需整齐排成一直线(图4-9-2,图4-10-8),但返折处不宜在伤口或骨隆突处。这种绷带包扎法容易松脱,不适用于关节部位。

(4)"8"字绷扎法:主要用于各关节。先在关节远侧环形绷扎几圈,然后斜向上越过关节,在关节近侧绕一圈。再向下越过关节,在关节下绕一圈。如此反复多次直至覆盖满意。关节都不包扎在内,除非用弹性绷带(图4-10-1~图4-10-6)。

(5)人字形绷扎法:主要用于两个粗细不同交界部位,如:腹股沟部、肩部或拇指部。这种包扎法对这些部位有很好的压迫作用(图4-11~图4-13)。

(6)回返绷扎法:主要用于指端、头部或残肢端,为一系列的左右或前后反折绷扎,直至该端全部遮盖后,再作环形绷扎固定(图4-14,图4-15)。

5. 三角巾包扎　三角巾在急救中的用途最广。一般由可洗的棉布制成,也可以用一次性使用的纸制成。摊开的三角巾可用作吊带,也可以用作敷料。

6. 套筒型绷带包扎　这种绷带有各种不同的尺寸。大的套筒绷带可以用于关节或将敷料固定于局部,小的套筒绷带可用于手指或足趾外伤的包扎。每种尺寸的套筒绷带都配备有相应的"上绷器"(applicator),固定的最好办法是用带子。

(1)套筒型绷带的裁剪长度是拟绷手指或足趾长度的2.5倍,然后将剪下的套筒型绷带放到"上绷器"上。

(2)将敷料放在伤口上。将"上绷器"上的套筒型绷带下拉至手指或足趾上。

(3)在手指或足趾的基部捏住套筒型绷带下段和纱布,向上撤除"上绷器",用一层纱布覆盖手指或足趾。

7. 绷带包扎的一般注意事项

(1)绷带包扎要注意平服美观。绷带包扎的外观是判断绷带包扎者熟练程度的重要指标之一。判断绷带包扎者水平的其他指标是包扎的目的是否已经达到,一段时间后位置是否有移动,以及病人是否舒适。绷带包扎要求贴身,又不能太紧(在去除绷带后皮肤上不遗留压痕)。

(2) **绷带包扎时不要打褶**。为了保证绷带的平服,必要时可以反折180°做人字形包扎(弹性绷带不必做人字形包扎)。在包扎过程中,保持绷带卷运行的力量适度。运行中坠落绷带卷提示心理素质不过硬,由于绷带松了,你不得不重新来。

(3) 由于纱布绷带存在网孔,能透气,因此,在固定时不要用胶布将网孔全部盖住。自粘绷带的固定比较简单,只需要固定其末端即可。用纱布绷带包扎四肢时,用于固定绷带的**胶布最好采用螺旋形粘贴**,以免影响肢体的血供。只要能满足**平服包扎**的要求,应该选用最宽的绷带,如:2.5 cm宽的绷带仅用于手指,5 cm宽的绷带用于手部和头部,其他部位基本都可以用7.5 cm宽的绷带。当然,足趾和足可以分别用2.5 cm或5 cm宽的绷带。

(4) 弹性绷带包扎时不能拉至弹性承受极限,否则就成普通绷带了。在用弹性绷带包扎四肢时,应该在远端紧些,近端松些。绷带不宜过紧,以去除绷带后皮肤上不遗留压痕为度。用弹性绷带包扎下肢时,应该将足趾包扎在内,否则足趾会肿胀。对于需要加压包扎的创口,可以在伤口上另加一些敷料,包扎也可以紧一些。不过,此时应该经常检查伤肢,以免血供受影响。

(5) 绷带会阻断肢体的血供,尤其当肢体有损伤水肿时。因此,绷扎时指端或趾端最好能露在外面,以便观察该肢体的血循环情况是否良好。应用卷带后发现有肢体疼痛、肿胀、青紫、麻木等症状时应立即追究原因,必要时解除或剪开绷带。

(6) 一般自内向外,并自远心端向躯干绷扎。绷扎开始必须先做两周环形绷扎,以固定绷带。患肢应保持在功能位(图4-16),如肘关节应屈曲90°。

Session 5　Basic cardiopulmonary resuscitation（CPR）

【Goals & requirements】

1. The intention of watching video tape or film is to provide students with the ability to further their knowledge in the specific field of cardiopulmonary resuscitation（CPR） without losing the overview of general theoretical and practical problems. The student will learn not only the proper medical procedures necessary for successful treatment in an emergency situation，but also the fundamental patho-physiology involved.

2. Correctly master the estimating skills such as accessing airways or taking accurate pulse checks.

3. Master the skills of basic life support（BLS）by practicing the techniques on CPR simulator，mouth-to-mouth ventilation and external chest compression.

4. Be familiar with the use of defibrillator（placement of the defibrillator paddles and caution）

5. Learn the skills of tracheal intubation by practicing on simulator.

【Progress schedule】

1. Watching video or film first.

2. Educator will demonstrate the techniques of CPR，and then students will be asked to follow step by step on CPR model or simulator.

3. At the end，educator will present his/her comment.

【Topics of this session】

A. Basic life support for cardiopulmonary arrest

Cardiac arrest may occur in a patient in any part of the hospital. The limiting factor in successful treatment of cardiac arrest is the short interval during which the cells of the brain can survive without oxygen. **If circulation and oxygen transport to the brain is not re-established in 4 to 6 minutes，the patient will suffer irreversible brain damage** and，in the majority of instances，death. It is unnecessary to listen for faint sounds in the chest. Time is better spent in re-establishing an airway and circulation.

To save the victim with cardiopulmonary arrest，all you need is two hands and a mouth.

Step 1：Gently shake the victim's shoulders and ask loudly："Are you all right?" if a casualty is unresponsive, shout for help and start CPR.

Step 2: Position the victim　Place the unconscious patient face up (extended supine position) on flat firm surface. Control the head and neck while turning the patient, especially if trauma is suspected.

Step 3: A (airway opening)　Establishing a patent, secure airway is the first step. In most instances the arrest is brought on by anoxia which is usually due to some obstruction of the airway, such as the tongue falls posteriorly, aspiration of vomitus, secretions, or blood, and foreign body in the pharynx. If the victim has no cervical spine injury, opening and maintaining an airway is best achieved by head tilt, chin lift and mouth open method (Fig. 5-1). Rescuers should use the finger sweep in the unconscious patient with a suspected airway obstruction only if solid material is visible in the oropharynx.

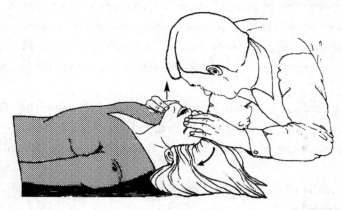

Fig. 5-1　Opening the airway by head tilt, chin lift and mouth opening maneuver
图 5-1　抬首—举颏—张口三步气道开放法

Uncooperative and combative patients should be assumed hypoxic, under the influence of drugs and/or alcohol, or to have suffered significant head injury. When in doubt definitive control of the airway using an endotracheal tube is appropriate.

Step 4: B (breathing)　Once the airway is open, check for signs of adequate spontaneous breath. Put one ear close to the victim's mouth, **feel** for exhaled airflow on your ear, **look** for rhythmic chest and abdominal movement, and **listen** for exhaled breath sounds at the nose and mouth.

In the first few minutes after cardiac arrest, a victim may be barely breathing, or taking infrequent, noisy gasps. Do not confuse this with normal breathing. Look, listen, and feel for no more than 10 seconds to determine whether the victim is breathing normally. If you have any doubt whether breathing is normal, act as if it is not normal.

If there is no sign of breathing, begin mouth-to-mouth ventilation immediately. While holding the jaw forward with one hand, tilt the head backward and pinch the nostrils closed with the other hand to prevent leakage of air through the nose. Take a deep breath; place your mouth tightly over the patient's and blow forcefully into his lungs (Fig. 5-2). When the chest has expanded adequately, remove your mouth from the patient's so that he can exhale. Blow 2 slow breaths into the victim without allowing time for the lungs to deflate fully when initiating resuscitation, and then repeat 2 artificial ventilations for every 30 chest compressions until other means of ventilation are available.

For mouth-to-mouth ventilation with exhaled air or bag-valve-mask(Fig. 5-3) ventilation with room air or oxygen, it is reasonable to give each breath within a 1-second inspiratory time to achieve chest rise, as severe gastric distention will markedly increase the risk of vomiting or regurgitation, with subsequent aspiration. After an advanced airway (e.g., tracheal tube or laryngeal mask airway) is placed, ventilate the patient's lungs with supplementary oxygen to make the chest rise. During CPR for a patient with an advanced airway in place, it is reasonable to ventilate the lungs at a rate of 8 to 10 ventilations per minute without pausing during chest compressions to deliver ventilations.

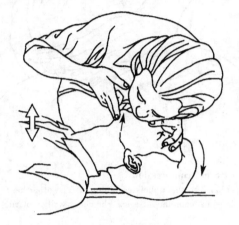

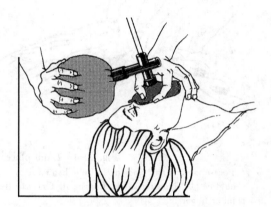

Fig. 5-2　Mouth-to-mouth ventilation
图 5-2　口对口人工呼吸

Fig. 5-3　Bag-valve-mask ventilation
图 5-3　呼吸囊—活瓣—面罩装置人工呼吸器

Sometimes during artificial ventilation air enters the stomach instead of the lungs. This condition is called gastric distension. It can be relieved by moderate pressure exerted with a flat hand between the navel and the rib cage. Before applying pressure, turn the victim's head to the side to prevent choking of the stomach contents that are often brought up during the process.

Step 5: C (circulation)　To assess circulation, two fingers are placed over the larynx and slid toward the rescuer into the groove between the trachea and the sternocleidomastoid muscle to attempt to palpate the carotid pulse. If no pulse is palpated, a proper method of external chest compression (cardiac massage or cardiac compression) should be initiated.

The closed-chest method should always be used until an endotracheal tube, a ventilation machine, and proper help have arrived. If the patient is not in a hospital, or if you are alone and there is doubt that you will be able to get help rapidly, the closed method is the only method.

The patient should be fully supine and lay on a firm surface, typically the floor or on a backboard. The rescuer stands or kneels at right angles to the patient, and places the heel of one hand with the heel of the other on top of it on the sternum, just cephalad to the xiphoid process (Fig. 5-4). Interlock the fingers of your hands and ensure that pressure is not applied over the victim's ribs. Do not apply any pressure over the upper abdomen or the bottom end of the bony sternum. Keep your arms straight and your shoulders directly over the patient's sternum. Use the weight of your upper body to achieve adequate depth of compression (Fig. 5-5). Sufficient pressure should be exerted to move the sternum at least 5 cm toward the vertebral column. After each compression, release all the pressure on the chest without losing contact between your hands and the sternum and allow complete recoil of the chest. Compression and release should take equal amounts of time.

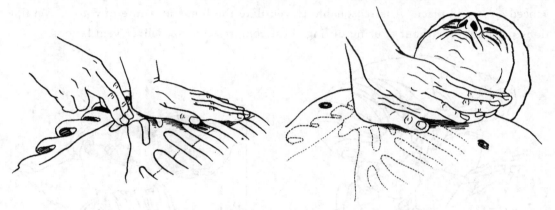

Fig. 5-4 Hand placement for external compression

Locate xiphoid and place heel of one hand 2 finger-breadths cephalad to the xiphoisternal notch. The other hand should be placed on top of the first hand. Only the heel of the bottom hand should touch the chest wall—not the palm or fingers.

图 5-4 心脏按压位置的快速确定法

沿季肋摸到剑突,选择剑突与胸骨交界线的头侧两横指处为按压点。将一手掌跟部置于按压点,另一手掌跟部重叠于前者之上。手指向上方翘起,仅掌根部与胸壁接触,手掌和手指不接触。

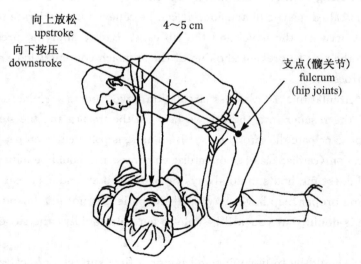

Fig. 5-5 The proper method of external chest compression

图 5-5 心脏按压姿势

If two or more persons are present, one should give massage to the heart at a rate of at least 100 compressions per minute while another gives mouth-to-mouth respiration by alternate positive-pressure ventilation— 30 compressions to 2 ventilations（Fig. 5-6）. Two or more rescuers should change the compressor role approximately every 2 minutes to prevent compressor fatigue and deterioration in quality and rate of chest compressions. When only one person is present in case of an arrest, attention should be concentrated on the massage: provide 30 compressions followed by 2 ventilations（30 : 2）. There is no question as to the adequacy of the circulation if a peripheral pulse is palpable. The absence of a palpable peripheral pulse is most likely due to improper massage.

Although it used to be follow your A-B-C（airway, breathing and chest compressions）, now, the 2010 CPR Guidelines want untrained lay rescuers to do **Hands Only CPR** on adult victims（taking C-A-B insteading of A-B-C to restart circulation earlier）who collapse（mostly from sudden cardiac arrest）in front of them. What cardiac arrest victims really need is for brain blood to get flowing again. When rescuers are worried about opening the airway and making an adequate seal, plus the "ick" factor and possibly digging a CPR mask out of a purse or briefcase, the delay can be significant. All that extra time is getting in the way of real help: Chest compressions.

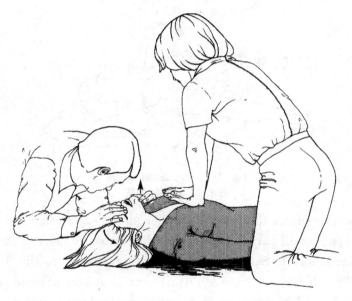

Fig. 5-6　Postioning for 2-rescuer CPR
Ventilator and compressor should be on opposite sides of victims
图 5-6　双人心肺复苏法
人工呼吸者与心脏按压者的位置相对

Step 6: D（defibrillation）　Some hearts begin to fibrillate. This is an unsatisfactory contraction and must be corrected by stopping the heart and re-establishing a normal beat. This is most commonly accomplished by electrical defibrillation.

Strengthening the chain of survival in emergency cardiac care, which is comprised of early access, early CPR, early defibrillation and early advanced care, is the most important way to improve the outcomes of sudden death patients. Early defibrillation is the key manner in which to save patients with cardiovascular diseases presenting with life-threatening ventricular arrhythmia. Early defibrillation for the witnessed ventricular fibrillation (VF) carries high survival rate of more than 90%. Each minute of delay when treating VF leads to a 7%~8% reduction of survival.

Precardial thump is indicated for adult patients with monitored cardiac arrest. Chest thump defibrillation may be especially useful in victims of high-voltage electrocution. The thump is administered sharply as a blow that uses the ulnar aspect of the clenched fist (Fig. 5-7) and is delivered from a point 25~30 cm above the chest.

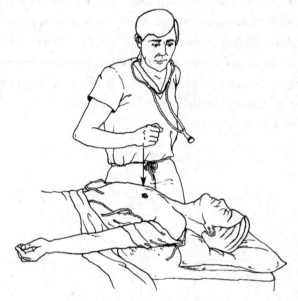

Fig. 5-7   Precardial thump
图 5-7   胸前捶击法

Defibrillation procedure: ①Victims should be placed supine on a firm surface; ②Ask someone else to apply conductive jelly to the paddles or use conductive pads; ③Switch on the monitor/defibrillator; ④Select an adequate energy level, usually 3 J/kg or 200 J; ⑤Press "Charge" to charge capacitor; ⑥Ensure paddles placement on the chest wall in the anterior-apex location; ⑦Be sure to warn everyone involved before applying shock, so that no one is touching the victim or the bed without intervening electrical insulation. Call "All clear"; ⑧Deliver shock by pressing both paddle discharge buttons simultaneously.

Caution: CPR effort should not be interrupted for more than a few seconds while defibrillation is being administered. Do not interrupt CPR while searching for defibrillation machine, paddles, or saline pads or adjusting the instrument. All of these tasks should be performed by others while cardiac compression continues. For most adults, administer 200 J of

DC countershock with one paddle electrode to the right of the sternum in the second or third interspace and the other paddle at the cardiac apex （Fig. 5-8）. Apply firm pressure on paddles diminishing transthoracic resistance. If one shock fails to eliminate VF, the VF may be of low amplitude and the incremental benefit of another shock is low. In such patients, immediate resumption of CPR, particularly effective chest compressions, is likely to confer a greater value than an immediate second shock.

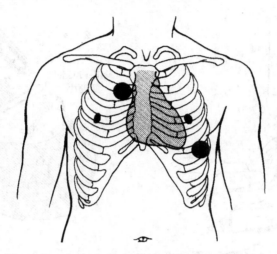

Fig. 5-8　Contact points for defibrillation electrodes.
Place one defibrillator paddle at aortic position and the apex electrode should be placed to the left of the nipple, with the centre of the electrode in the midaxillary line.
图 5-8　除颤电极安放位置
一个电极放在右锁骨下窝,另一个电极放在左乳头外侧腋中线处。

B. Basic techniques of tracheal intubation.

1. Equipment　The tip of the endotracheal tube should be lubricated with lidocaine jelly, and a stylet should be inserted. The endotracheal balloon should be tested to assure patency. There are two types of laryngoscope blades, the straight （Miller） and curved （Macintosh） blades. Individual preference usually guides blade choice.

2. Patient preparation　One of the most important aspects of the technique is proper patient positioning. Alignment of the oral, pharyngeal, and laryngeal axes is accomplished by placing the patient in the sniffing position. Preoxygenation can be attained with a bag-valve-mask device or a 100% oxygen mask in the breathing patient.

3. Intubation technique　After patient positioning is attained, endotracheal intubation is attempted. The laryngoscope is held in the left hand and inserted into the right side of the patient's mouth, displacing the tongue to the left. The straight blade is inserted over the epiglottis whereas the curved blade is inserted in the vallecula. With the blade in place, force is directed upward and away from the body （in the direction of the handle） in

a plane 45 degrees from horizontal to expose the vocal cords (Fig. 5-9). The handle should neither be used with a prying motion nor the upper teeth used as a fulcrum. The endotracheal tube is inserted in the right corner of the mouth and advanced under direct vision through the vocal cords until the proximal end of the cuff is below the cords. Attempts at intubation should last no more than 2 minutes. Bag-valve-mask ventilation and reoxygenation for 2 to 3 minutes should occur between attempts.

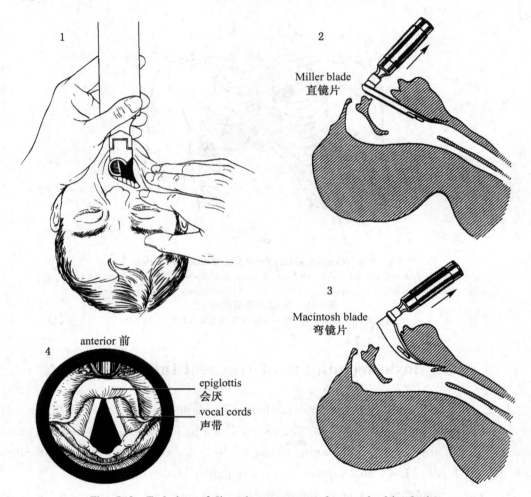

Fig. 5-9　Technique of direct laryngoscopy and orotracheal intubation.
　1. The straight laryngoscope blade is passed behind the tongue and deep to the tip of the epiglottis. 2. Lateral view showing straight laryngoscope blade deep to the tip of epiglottis exposing glottic opening. 3. Lateral view showing that the tip of the curved laryngoscope blade is inserted anterior to the epiglottis, between the epiglottis and the base of the tongue. 4. View of glottis as seen through a laryngoscope with a curved blade.

图 5-9　直接喉镜下经口气管插管
　1. 插入直镜片喉镜,将舌推向左侧,将会厌挑起;2. 直镜片喉镜插入的侧面观,将会厌挑起显露声门裂;3. 弯镜片喉镜插入的侧面观,喉镜片的尖端位于会厌前方,即会厌与舌根部之间;4. 弯喉镜下所见到的声门裂。

实习五　心肺复苏基本技术

【目的和要求】

1. 通过放教学电影和电视录像,较全面、系统地复习心肺复苏技术和基本知识。不仅要学习现场急救的要点,还需要了解相关的病理生理基础。

2. 掌握心跳呼吸骤停的诊断。

3. 通过训练模型练习,掌握基本生命支持(口对口人工呼吸和胸外心脏按压)的要领。

4. 熟悉电除颤器的用法(电极的放置和注意事项)。

5. 在训练模型上学习气管插管,使操作熟练。

【实习程序】

1. 先观看教学电影、电视录像。

2. 示教后,再用训练模型练习心肺复苏。

3. 结束前,教师点评、小结。

【实习项目】

一、心跳呼吸骤停时的基本生命支持

心脏骤停在医院的任何场所都可能发生。心肺骤停救治难以成功的主要因素是脑细胞在无氧环境下的生存时间很短,**如果循环和氧输送在 4～6 分钟不能重建,脑细胞就会发生不可逆的损害**,其中大多数人会死亡。因此,不应该把时间花在听诊有无心音上,而应该抓紧时间重建气道和循环。

抢救心跳呼吸骤停病人,只需要一双手和一张嘴。

第一步:呼叫请求帮助

边轻摇病人肩部,边呼唤病人"您怎么啦",观察有无反应。若无反应,立即呼救请求帮助并着手 CPR。

第二步:放好体位

将病人摆放成仰卧位(面朝上),转动体位时要注意保护头颈部,尤其当疑有创伤时。

第三步:A(airway opening)开放气道

首先要做的是保持气道通畅。心搏呼吸骤停病人通常存在一定程度的气道阻塞,常见原因有:后坠的舌根、呼吸道分泌物、血块、口腔异物堵塞气道。若病人无颈椎损伤,应先用手法(三步气道开放法)开放气道(图 5-1),即:抬首(头后仰)、举颏(抬下颌)、张口。对神志不清、疑有呼吸道梗阻的病人,仅当见到口咽部固体异物时,需要用手指抠出气道内的堵塞物。

第四步：B(breathing)正压通气

开放气道后，检查病人有无自主呼吸。检查时将耳贴近病人口部，**感觉**病人的呼气，同时**看看**病人胸廓有无起伏、**听听**口鼻有无呼吸音。

在心脏骤停的最初几分钟，病人可以偶有呼吸或喘气声，千万不要误认为是正常呼吸。通过看、听和感觉来判断病人有无呼吸，时间不要超过 10 秒。如果你不能确定呼吸是否正常，请看作呼吸不正常来处理。

若无自主呼吸，应立即进行口对口人工呼吸。先将病人的头置于"三步气道开放"位置，术者一手抬下颌，另一手保持病人头部后仰，同时以拇指和食指捏闭病人鼻孔防止漏气。深吸一口气，用自己的嘴将病人的口封闭，用力将气体吹入(图 5-2)。首次操作时，可连续缓慢吹入 2 次，然后以每 30 次胸外心脏按压 2 次人工呼吸的频率进行。

无论是用呼出气做口对口人工呼吸，还是用室内空气做呼吸囊—活瓣—面罩装置(图 5-3)呼吸，每次吹气时间不宜超过 1 秒，见有胸廓抬起即可。严重胃扩张可导致内容物反流和误吸。在高级气道(气管插管或喉罩)建立后，即可用氧气进行通气。此时，通气频率在 8～10 次/分钟即可。通气时，不要停止心脏按压。

人工通气的气体可以进入胃内，造成胃扩张。此时，可以将病人的头偏向一侧防止吐出物造成的窒息，用一只手在脐与胸廓间适度施压来缓解胃扩张。

第五步：C(circulation)胸外心脏按压

评估循环状态的基本方法是将食、中两指放在喉前，然后，向侧方滑至胸锁乳突肌内侧沟处扪颈动脉搏动。如果扪不到颈动脉搏动，就应该开始恰当的胸外心脏按压(心脏按摩)。

在医院外，在没有气管插管、呼吸机和其他高级复苏手段的条件下，病人有需要紧急救护时，胸外心脏按压是基础。

病人平卧，背部垫一木板或平卧于地板上。术者立于或跪于病人一侧。沿季肋摸到剑突，选择剑突与胸骨交界线的头侧两横指处为按压点(图 5-4)。不要压在肋骨上，也不要压在胸骨下端。将一手掌跟部置于按压点，另一手掌跟部重叠于前者之上。手指向上方翘起，两臂伸直(肩在胸骨的正上方)，凭自身重力通过双臂和双手掌，垂直向胸骨加压(图 5-5)，使胸骨至少下陷 5 cm，然后立即放松，但双手不离开胸壁，使胸廓自行恢复原位。如此反复操作，按压与松开时间比为 1:1。

双人或多人复苏时，心脏按压的频率至少是 100 次/分，每按压 15 次进行口对口人工呼吸 2 次(图 5-6)。心脏按压每 2 分钟应换人，防止因疲劳而影响复苏效果。复苏时主要精力应放在心脏按压上：每做心脏按压 30 次进行口对口人工呼吸 2 次(30:2)。心脏按压有效时可触及颈动脉或股动脉的搏动，扪不到周围脉搏往往提示按压手法不当。

尽管经典的复苏程序是 A－B－C[airway(气道)、breathing(呼吸)和胸外按压(chest compressions)]，不过，2010 CPR 指南要求非医疗专业的施救人员对突然倒在你面前的成年遇难者(这些人大多是心脏骤停病人)**仅做手工复苏**(用 C-A-B 取代 A-B-C，目的是尽早重启循环)。因为心脏骤停病人所需要的就是重新获得大脑血液灌注。当施救者为气道开放和口对口呼吸犹豫不决时(不可否认对非医疗专业的施救人员来讲，口对口呼吸会"给人带来不快"；寻找面罩也会花费时间)，这就会拖延 CPR。你可以将这些时间利用起来做实实在在的急救：胸外按压。

第六步：D(defibrillation)心脏电除颤　　心脏颤动是一种无效收缩,必须纠正,恢复正常心律。最常用的手段是电除颤。

心脏急救"生命链"的重要环节包括早呼救、早 CPR、早除颤和早高级生命支持。对室性心律失常危及生命的病人来说,早除颤就成了救命的关键步骤。对这种病人,早除颤可以挽救 90%以上的病人;随着时间的推移,除颤成功的机会迅速下降,每耽搁 1 分钟成功率下降7%～8%。

对成人突发性心搏骤停病人,特别是高压电击伤病人,最初目击者,可给予一次胸前捶击。胸前捶击的方法:术者握拳,距胸部 25～30 cm 高,用小鱼际侧对病人胸部正中(胸骨中段)用力捶击一次(图 5-7)。

除颤步骤如下:①置病人于平卧位;②手控电极涂专用导电胶;③开启除颤器;④选择能量,首次除颤以 3 J/kg(约 200 J);⑤除颤器充电;⑥两电极正确放置于胸前和心尖部;⑦确定无周围人员直接或间接与病人接触,此称"清空";⑧同时按压两个放电按钮进行电击。

注意:电除颤时,CPR 不宜停顿数秒。不要因寻找除颤器、电极或调制仪器而停止CPR。所有这些工作都应该由其他人员完成,保证 CPR 不间断。对大多数成人来说,用200 J 直流电即可。位置对除颤和心脏复律极为重要。一般用前侧位,前电极放在胸骨右缘第 2、3 肋间,侧电极放在心尖部(图 5-8)。电极必须涂导电胶紧压于胸壁,减小电阻。如果一次电击未能复律,其原因可能是低幅心室颤动,增加能量再次电击复律的可能性很小。此时,应该继续 CPR,特别是胸外按压。

二、气管插管技术

物品准备:气管导管尖端应涂润滑剂,插入管芯。检查充气套囊是否漏气。喉镜镜片有直和弯两种,取决于各人的喜好。

病人准备:最重要的一点是把病人放在头过伸、后仰体位,使口、咽、喉成一直线。用呼吸囊—活瓣—面罩装置做加压纯氧人工呼吸。

插管:病人体位摆好后,即可进行插管。术者左手持喉镜从病人口的右侧进入,把舌推向左侧。用直镜片时需要越过会厌将会厌挑起,弯镜片插入会厌谷即可。然后,左手持镜柄与水平线呈 45°角(沿镜柄方向)上提显露声门裂(图 5-9),此时,喉镜切勿以上门齿为支点上撬。显露声门后,在直视下,右手持气管导管从右口角轻柔地插入,至套囊进入声门下为止。遇有插管困难,显露喉头逾 2 分钟者当暂停操作,用呼吸囊—活瓣—面罩装置行加压氧吸入 2～3 分钟,再继续试插管。

Session 6 Basic surgical skills for laparoscopic surgery

【Goals & requirements】

1. General surgical principles: entry into the abdomen, handling of the instruments during the procedure.

2. By box trainer-based education module, be familiar with methods of grasping tissue, picking and placing, and handling of objects between instruments, pattern cutting, placement of a ligating loop, suture, intracorporeal and extracorporeal knot tying under laparoscopic environment.

【Progress schedule】

1. Students are divided into small working groups (2 students a group). Educator introduces a simulator-based training program, traditional box trainers or virtual reality (VR) surgical simulators.

2. Educator will demonstrate the commonly used techniques in laparoscopic surgery first, and then students will be asked to follow step by step.

3. Watching video or film.

4. At the end, educator will present his/her comment.

【Topics of this session】

In vivo simulations of exercises are often instantiated into **box trainers** with inanimate objects, such as string, needles, beans, cloth, and latex tubing. Nine different tasks designed to improve **hand-eye coordination** and to stimulate **psychomotor skills** constitute the basis of this system. The complexity of these tasks ranges from basic grasping targets to transferring them between instruments to performing these tasks with an increased difficulty level, including suture and the use of diathermy.

A. Instruments and Telescopes

1. 10-mm, 0-degree telescope
2. 5-mm, 0-degree telescope
3. Veress needle and reducer
4. Two 5-mm laparoscopic graspers and one needle holder
5. Laparoscopic suction/irrigation device

6. Electrocautery hook and spatula，or electrocautery scissors

7. Laparoscopic surgical clips

B.　Fundamental skills for laparoscopic surgery

1. Manipulation angle　Ideal positioning of the needle holder and the assisting forceps is a 60 degrees to 90 degrees angle and set 15 cm apart to avoid a "chopstick effect". The ideal port position for closure of a choledochotomy spreads the needle holder and assisting forceps by 60 degrees to 90 degrees with one-half of the instrument (15 cm) in the patient and one-half out (Fig. 6-1).

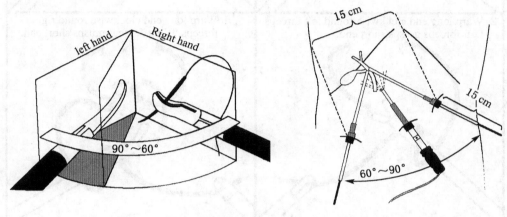

Fig. 6-1　Manipulation angle
图 6-1　理想操作角

2. Grasping-and-placing exercises　Grasp beans with graspers and place them into a plastic bag or a cylinder hold by another hand.

3. Grasping-and-transferring exercises　Grasp stitch with grasper and arm it on needle holder as you wish.

4. Grasping-clipping-cutting exercises　Grasp，clip and cut cloth on which vessels are drawn to mimic mesenteric vessel cutting.

5. Pattern cutting exercises　Cut cloth or paper.

6. Intracorporeal knot tying exercises　Use forceps to practice instrument tie intracorporeally：

(1) Laparoscopic reef knot/square knot：Print out the Instruction diagram (Fig. 6-2) and paste it onto the front of a cardboard. This diagram will enable you to learn the moves of laparoscopic knot tying. Then punch 2 holes in the lower border of the cardboard. Pass a cord through the holes as in the diagram. Follow the instructions on the diagram using laparoscopic needle holders.

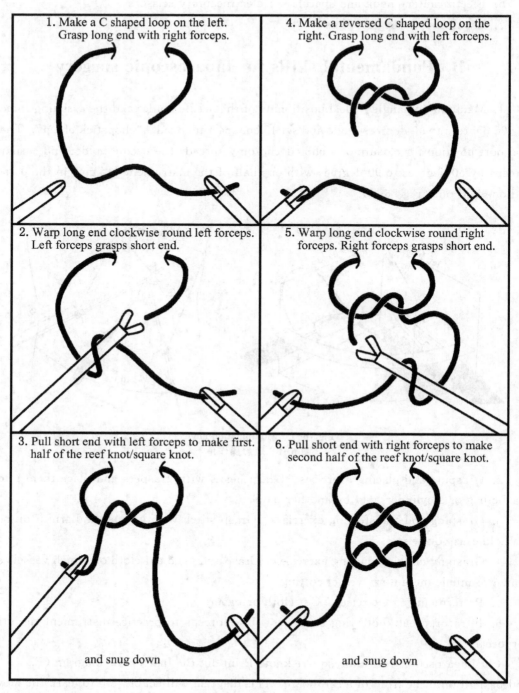

1. Make a C shaped loop on the left. Grasp long end with right forceps.

4. Make a reversed C shaped loop on the right. Grasp long end with left forceps.

2. Warp long end clockwise round left forceps. Left forceps grasps short end.

5. Warp long end clockwise round right forceps. Right forceps grasps short end.

3. Pull short end with left forceps to make first half of the reef knot/square knot.

and snug down

6. Pull short end with right forceps to make second half of the reef knot/square knot.

and snug down

Fig. 6-2　Intracorporeal reef knot/square knot
图 6-2　体内打方结

（2）Intracorporeal Aberdeen knot tying（Fig. 6-3）

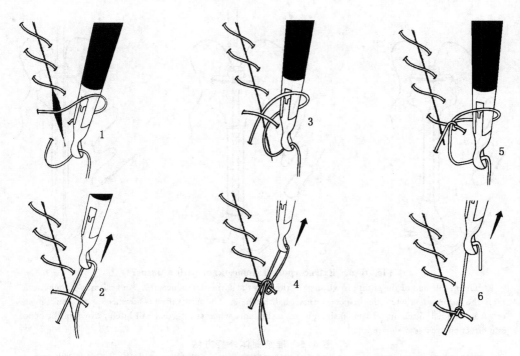

Fig. 6-3　Intracorporeal Aberdeen knot tying used for termination of running suture line

图 6-3　腹腔镜下的 Aberdeen 结（用于连续缝合完毕时）

7. Extracorporeal knot tying exercises：

(1) Making knot by a ligating loop (Fig. 6-4)

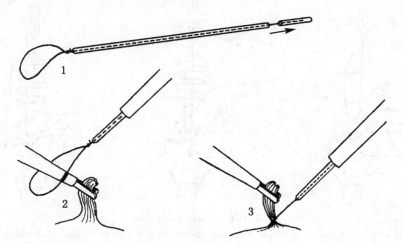

Fig. 6-4　Preformed knot

1. Preformed loop ligature. The end piece is pulled in the direction of the arrow to tighten the ligature；2. After lassoing the grasping instruments，the pedicle is isolated；3. The loop is slid to proper position and tightened.

图 6-4　套结器打结

1. 将套结器的尾部折断，按箭头方向抽拉收紧；2. 通过抓钳套住组织；3. 将线收紧至适当位置。

(2) Making knot by a knot pusher (Fig. 6-5)

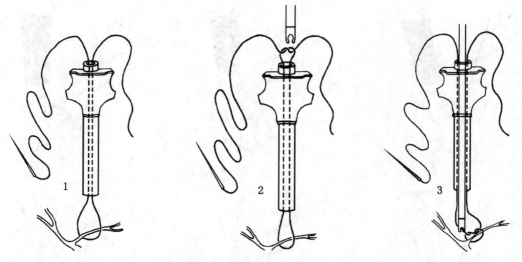

Fig. 6-5 Extracorporeal square knot with a pusher

1. The needle end of the suture is withdrawn through the suture introducer; 2. An assistant's finger separates the suture ends while the surgeon forms a half hitch; 3. The first throw is advanced with a knot pusher. A second half hitch in the same fashion forms a slipknot, whereas a second half hitch thrown in the opposite direction creates a square knot.

图 6-5 推结器体外打方结

1. 将缝线的针端拖出套管针；2. 助手用手指将线的两端分开，术者先打一个半结；3. 用推结器将这个半结推入，再打第二个半结形成滑结，但要按相反方向推结使之形成方结。

（3）Making sliding knots：The common used sliding knots are fisherman's knot (Fig. 6-6) and Roeder knot (Fig. 6-7)

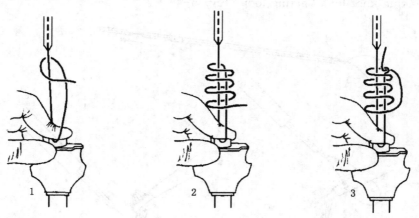

Fig. 6-6 Fisherman's knot

1. After suturing, both ends of the suture are withdrawn and separated by an assistant's finger; 2. Hold both sutures between the thumb and index finger and throw three to four successive loops around the post with the first around your thumb creating a loop; 3. Pass the free end of the long suture through the initial loop made by your thumb and tighten the knot configuration by pulling the loop (long) limb. A series of half hitches on alternating posts (total of 3 or 4) will secure the fisherman's knot.

图 6-6 渔夫结的打法

1. 缝合完成后，缝线的两端从打孔器(Trocar)中抽出、分开；2. 用拇指和食指捏住线的两头，将长的线头绕两根线3～4圈，但第一圈要绕过拇指形成一个线襻；3. 将长线头的尾端穿过该线襻，收紧成结。若能再打几个半结(3～4 个)可以防止结滑脱。

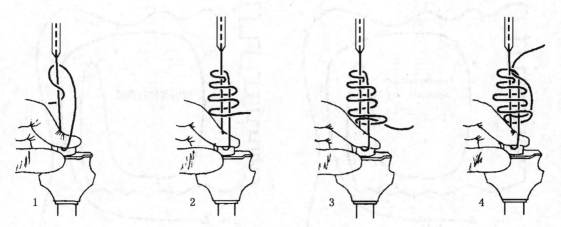

Fig. 6-7　Roeder knot

1. After suturing, both ends of the suture are withdrawn and separated by an assistant's finger; 2. A half hitch is formed; 3. Three wraps around both suture ends are made before inserting the long end through the last loop; 4. The long end may also be inserted through the initial loop.

图 6-7　Roeder 结的打法

1. 缝合完成后,缝线的两端从打孔器(Trocar)中抽出、分开;2. 先打一个半结;3. 左手抓住半结和一个线头,右手将另一个线头绕两根线三圈,然后穿过最后一个圈;4. 也可以再穿过第一个圈。

8. Suturing skill training: Suturing skills are practiced using standard sutures and needles through plastic drains or cadaveric tissue specimens (Fig. 6-1).

9. Practice dissection and electrocautery through cadaveric tissue specimens. Understand the principles and hazards of electrocautery.

C.　Performance evaluation

1. Aptitude Test　Print out the Fig. 6-8 and follow the instructions.

(1) Instructions: Use stitch scissors. Start the computer clock. Start cutting at the Start mark. Continue cutting along the black track until you reach the Finish sign. Stop the computer clock. Record your time.

(2) Add penalty times for: ①Straying outside the black line—10 seconds per event. ②Tearing the paper — 30 seconds per event. ③Add up your total score.

(3) Results: ①Less than 6 minutes **Good**. ②6 to 8 minutes **Average**. ③More than 8 minutes **Not so good**. You need more practice, or you may find the program and surgery too much for you.

2. Laparoscopic reef knot/square knot　3 reef knot/square knots in one minutes are considered **Average**.

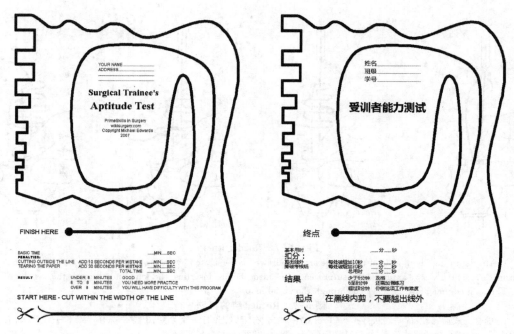

Fig. 6-8　Aptitude test
图 6-8　剪图测试

实习六　腹腔镜外科基本技术

【目的和要求】

1. 熟悉手术的一般原则：进腹、手术中的器械使用（熟悉安全建立气腹的方法和压力等）、病人的体位等。

2. 通过在盒式训练器中练习，熟悉腹腔镜外科基本技术：操纵摄像镜、抓取组织、抓取和放置物品、用器械交换物品、按要求剪纸剪线、套线、缝合和体内、外打结。

【实习程序】

1. 学生以 2 人为一小组。教师介绍盒式训练器或虚拟仿真手术模拟器。

2. 教师示教后，学生练习腹腔镜外科基本技术：抓取组织、抓取和放置物品、用器械传递物品、按要求剪物品、套线、缝合和体内、外打结。

3. 观看教学电影和电视录像。

4. 结束后，教师点评、小结。

【实习项目】

腹腔镜的活体模拟训练常用**盒式训练器**，盒式训练器内准备了缝线、缝针、大豆、布和胶管等实物。本实验包含了 9 项难度不同的操作，从简单地抓取物品、用器械传递物品，到复杂的缝合和电凝，目的是训练操作者**手眼协调能力**和**心理运动技能**。

一、腹腔镜常用器械

1. 10-mm，0-度镜

2. 5-mm，0-度镜

3. Veress 气腹针和转换器

4. 5-mm 腹腔镜抓钳 2 把，5-mm 腹腔镜持针器 1 把

5. 腹腔镜吸引器和冲洗器

6. 电凝钩、电铲和电剪

7. 腹腔镜钛夹

二、腹腔镜外科基本技术

1. 理想操作角　持针器与辅助抓钳之间的夹角最好能在 60°～90°，两把杆子相距 15 cm 左右，避免"同轴效应"。缝合胆总管切口时，持针器与辅助抓钳之间的夹角最好能在 60°～90°，器械长度的一半（15 cm）在病人体内，一半在病人体外（图 6-1）。

2. 抓—放练习　用抓钳抓取大豆后将大豆放入塑料袋内或圆筒内。

3. 抓—传练习　用器械抓取缝针,并能用抓钳协助,根据需要调整缝针在持针器上的位置。

4. 抓—夹—剪练习　在布上画肠系膜血管,然后,练习分离、钛夹钳夹、剪断,也可以用线绳练习。

5. 剪图练习　练习剪布或纸上的图案。

6. 腹腔镜手术体内打结

(1) 腹腔镜下方结的打法:将图6-2打印出来,贴在一块薄硬板纸上,在硬板纸的下端打两个孔,将该硬板纸放入训练盒内。将一根缝线穿过这两个孔。按照图6-2的步骤用抓钳或持针钳练习腔镜下器械打结。

(2) 腹腔镜下 Aberdeen 结的打法(图6-3)

7. 腹腔镜手术体外打结训练

(1) 用套结器打结(图6-4)。

(2) 在体外打方结后用推结器逐个推入腹腔打结(图6-5)。

(3) 打滑结:常用的滑结有渔夫结(图6-6)和 Roeder 结(图6-7)两种。

8. 缝合技术训练　用标准的缝针和缝线练习胶管的缝合,也可用离体组织练习缝合(图6-1)。

9. 分离技术(血管或神经)和电凝技术训练　用离体组织进行。并了解电凝的原理和危险。

三、能力评价

1. 双手协调能力测试　把图6-8打印出来,按说明进行操作。

(1) 说明:用线剪。开始计时。从"起点"标记处开始沿黑线剪开,直至"终点"标记。停止计时。计算耗时。

(2) 扣分标准:①剪出黑线外:每处加10秒。②撕破图案纸:每处加30秒。③计算总耗时。

(3) 结果判断:①耗时少于6分钟,为**良好**;②6～8分钟,为**及格**;③大于8分钟,为**不及格**,提示你需要多练,或该项目和外科不适合你。

2. 腹腔镜下打结测试　每分钟打3个方结为**及格**。

Session 7 Abdominal surgery demonstration on animal models（anaesthesia，venous cutdown，appendectomy，splenectomy，enterectomy and end-to-end anastomosis，and partial gastrectomy and gastrojejunal anastomosis）

【Goals & requirements】

1. To understand surgical approaches and incisions and the use of appropriate instruments

2. To know the materials and methods used for wound closure and anastomoses（sutures，knots and needles）

3. To know the techniques for skin and bowel closure and anastomoses

4. The hands-on training on animal model encompasses five learning sessions each four hours long. Students are encouraged to discuss anything that varies from the practice with their program director.

【Topics of this session】

1. See Session 8 for anaesthesia，venous cutdown，and appendectomy.

2. See Session 9 for splenectomy.

3. See Session 10 for enterectomy and end-to-end anastomosis.

4. See Session 12 for partial gastrectomy and gastrojejunal anastomosis.

实习七　动物腹部手术示教（麻醉、静脉切开、阑尾切除术、脾切除术、小肠部分切除对端吻合术和胃部分切除胃空肠吻合术）

【目的和要求】

1. 了解外科手术的入路，以及手术刀、血管钳、剪刀的应用。

2. 熟悉伤口缝合和吻合所需的材料（缝线、缝针）和方法。

3. 熟悉皮肤和肠管缝合的技巧。

4. 动物操作有 5 次实训机会，每次 4 小时，每个同学都有一次机会承担不同的手术团队角色。鼓励学生提前预习，遇到问题时，学生应该随时向老师请教，以保证手术顺利进行。

【实习项目】

1. 麻醉、静脉切开和阑尾切除术参见本书实习八。

2. 脾切除术参见本书实习九。

3. 小肠部分切除对端吻合术参见本书实习十。

4. 胃部分切除胃—空肠吻合术参见本书实习十二。

Session 8　Hands-on training on animal models （anaesthesia， venous cutdown or venopuncture， and appendectomy）

【Goals & requirements】

1. Experience performing an appendectomy procedure through the hands-on training program to train basic surgical skills and establish a good background of surgical skill for future clinical practice， rather than to complete a operation.

2. Enhance intraoperative aseptic techniques before performing procedures on real patients.

3. Learn anesthesia techniques and intravenous infusion skills in dogs. Enable trainees to work together as a team on an operation and try to have good communication with other team members.

【Progress schedule】

1. Students are divided into small working groups (5 students a group). Anesthetist is responsible for animal catching and restraint， anesthesia， venous cutdown， intravenous infusion， and making anesthesia note. The scrub nurse should wash hands first. The first assistant is responsible for skin prep of surgical field.

2. Students will be asked to preview appendectomy procedure and follow the instruction step by step to perform the operation. After the surgery is completed， soiled instruments should be washed， dried， and lubricated， and then the room should be cleaned.

3. After the session of hands-on training on animal models， surgeons are expected to dictate operative note and postoperative reports day by day until suture removal. These surgical documentations are kept in the Department of Surgery.

【Topics of this session】

A. Anesthesia & Venous Access

1. Please refer to **Course Overview** of this book for preoperative prep and anesthesia for dogs. Then assistant takes the unconscious dog on operation table.

2. Venous cutdown　Clinically venous cutdown is performed to gain emergency venous access when other sites are not available or when multiple intravenous lines are required. In dogs， the lateral saphenous vein in the hindlimb is the preferred site for a cutdown.

(1) Equipment: Assemble all of the necessary equipment， including the container of intravenous fluid and connecting tubing， and make sure that the tubing has been flushed to remove air.

Select a sterile plastic tube of adequate diameter. Cut the tube to form a short bevel catheter， but not too sharp. The catheter is attached to a 2 ml or 5 ml syringe filled with normal saline and flushed to remove air.

(2) The saphenous vein is located laterally on the hind leg 3 cm above the hock joint and is easier to see when the fur is shaved and the area wiped with alcohol (Fig. 8-1). With the dog on his side, brace one hand on the knee of his uppermost rear leg, to both control movement and to distend the vein.

(3) Sterilize and drape the skin of the area. Anesthetize the area with the 1% lidocaine. Omit this step if the dog has been anesthetized intraperitoneally.

(4) With the No. 15 scalpel blade, make a 2 cm superficial transverse incision transverse or parallel to the vein, being careful not to cut through the vein.

(5) A thumb forceps is held in the left hand and the skin of wound edge is grasped. Using a mosquito clamp, dissect the tissues in the long axis of the vein to isolate the vein about 1.5 cm. Pass the clamp under the vein and dissect the underlying tissue. Place two silk

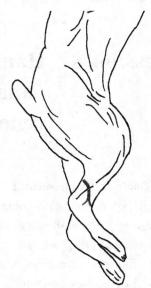

Fig. 8-1 The saphenous vein in
the dog hindlimb
图 8-1 大隐静脉的解剖位置

sutures around the vein. Tie the distal ligature, place it on gentle traction (Fig. 8-2).

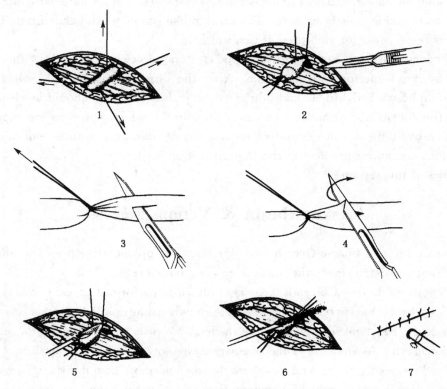

Fig. 8-2 Venous cutdown procedure
图 8-2 静脉切开术

(6) Perform a venotomy using a No. 11 scalpel blade with the blade in a horizontal position and pass the blade through the midportion of the vein. Then turn the cutting edge of the blade upward, and open the top of the vein. Take care not to transect the vein.

(7) Insert the catheter with bevel up, and pass it 10 cm proximally up the vein (it is unnecessary to pass it farther). Connect the intravenous tubing to the catheter, and begin the infusion. Tie the proximal ligature around the vein (which now encloses the catheter). Make it snug but not too tight, or it will cut through the vein, leaving the catheter loose.

(8) Suture the wound using a simple interrupted stitch. Secure the catheter to the skin with a skin stitch. The catheter is brought out through the skin separately from the main incision.

(9) When discontinuing fluid infusion, cut the suture securing the catheter before removing the catheter and applying pressure on the vessel to prevent bleeding.

3. Venopuncture　Clinically venopuncture is a commonly used operation for obtaining blood sample or administration of IV fluids during anesthesia and surgery. The marginal ear vein of the rabbit is useful for collection of small volumes of blood and may be used for intravenous injection.

(1) Equipment: A short bevel needle not more than 3 cm long and a syringe of 5 ml or 2 ml capacity are recommended. Butterfly infusion sets also work well. Prior to insertion of the butterfly or short bevel needle, the intravenous infusion system including drip chamber and the syringe should be precharged with normal saline or glucose solution.

(2) The marginal ear vein of rabbit is used almost exclusively for intravenous injection. The hair over the vein may be clipped or shaved and the skin cleansed with alcohol or alcohol-iodine before making the injection.

The vein can be distended by flicking the margin with the fingers for few times. Pinching off the vein near the base of the ear will also help to distend the vein. Nitroglycerin ointment also promotes vasodilation. Administration of 1 mg of Acepromazine to an adult rabbit facilitates restraint, reduces distress and dilates the marginal ear vein.

(3) The vein is occluded, the needle carefully inserted. The needle is inserted parallel to the vein and the tip directed into the lumen along the longitudinal axis. Then the needle is advanced slightly. Draw back. If blood appears in the hub of the needle, the drug may be injected. If not, try redirecting the needle (before you pull it out of the skin) and repeat. You may need to try several times while learning. Using a new, sharp needle for each stick, even if it is the same animal, will improve your chances for success. Once the needle is withdrawn, it is necessary to put pressure on the vessel to prevent bleeding.

Certain guidelines can be given, but only practice provides proficiency. Veins may be expected to roll, collapse, or shift, making entrance difficult. A precise, careful introduction of the needle is best and several attempts may be required. Starting at distal sites will allow repeat attempts more proximally.

B. Laparotomy

It should be the surgeon's aim to employ the type of incision considered to be the most suitable for particular operation about to be performed. Maingot's principles for a surgical incision are accessibility, extensibility and security. The choice of the incision depends on many factors: the organ to be investigated, surgeon's preference, whether speed is an essential consideration, the build of the patient, the degree of obesity and the presence of previous abdominal incisions.

In general, vertical incisions, median or paramedian, provide excellent and rapid access and can, if necessary, be extended the whole length of the abdomen to exploit all four quadrants. Transverse and oblique incisions have a better reputation for freedom from disruption.

（A）Access to abdomen by midline incision

1. After skin preparation, surgical field is squared off and draped.

2. The usual incision for the procedures is a midline xiphoumbilical incision some 10 cm long.

(1) Tips for skin incision: The surgeon holds the knife as holding table-knife (Fig. 2-8) and the scalpel is perpendicular to the skin surface. The knife passes through the stretched skin down to subcutaneous tissues but not at this stage through the line alba. An adequate force should be used when making the skin incision to avoid cutting several times.

(2) Tips for hemostasis: Hemostasis is one of basic surgical skills, which reduces blood loss and keeps the operation field clear. Hemostasis in the skin and subcutaneous tissues is obtained by the method of the surgeon's choice. The usual method is that the bleeding points are gently compressed by sponge, picked up by hemostatic clamps and then ligated. Since the clamped tissue will be destroyed, the tip of the clamp should grasp the end of the blood vessel, the tip of the vessel only and not the adjacent tissue. Each of the hemostatic clamps may also be touched with a diathermy point. The abdominal wall is incised and the hemostasis is carried out in layers.

(3) Tips for ligation: The classic method to make an assured hemostasis is to grasp bleeding point (the end of the blood vessel) using the tip of hemostatic clamps and then ligate the vessel with thread. After grasping the bleeding points, the assistant lifts the hemostatic clamp by holding the ring of the hemostat upward, when the surgeon passes a thread around the vessel at the tip of the hemostat. Then the assistant elevates the tip of the clamp by depressing the handle, when the surgeon makes the first half hitch. After the first half hitch is set, the assistant removes the hemostat; the first half hitch is tightened further before the second is begun. Once the knot has been securely tied, the ends

must be cut. Cutting sutures entails running the tips of the scissors lightly down the suture strand to the knot, turning the blade 45° and cutting. The ends are left approximately 3 mm from the knot, to decrease tissue reaction and minimize the amount of foreign material left in the wound (Fig. 2-39).

3. When the skin and subcutaneous tissues is incised, and hemostasis is completed, the wound should be protected from contamination by placing a fenestrated drape or two towels secured by Allis clamps.

The line alba is next incised in the line of the incision to expose the extraperitoneal fat and underlying diaphanous peritoneum.

4. When the surgeon holds a thumb forceps (or hemostatic clamp) in his left hand and the assistant holds a hemostatic clamp in his right hand, the peritoneum has been grasped at a point halfway from the xiphoid to the umbilicus. Then a small incision is being made in the peritoneum using a scalpel (Fig. 8-3). Before dividing the peritoneum, the surgeon, using the index finger and the thumb, must be sure that an abdominal viscus has not been grasped by the clamps. The thumb forceps and hemostatic clamp are replaced by another hemostatic clamp with which upward traction is applied to the peritoneum. The surgeon retracts with two fingers of the left hand in the abdominal cavity to protect the abdominal viscera and to permit the division of the peritoneum toward the xiphoid process or umbilicus using scissors (Fig. 8-4).

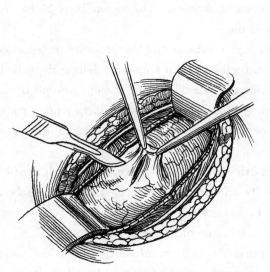

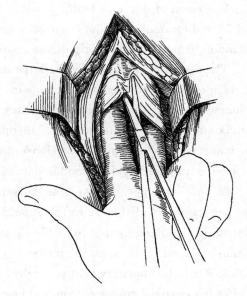

Fig. 8-3　The peritoneum is grasped at a point halfway by two hemostatic clamps

图 8-3　两人交替钳夹腹直肌后鞘和腹膜，然后切开

Fig. 8-4　The surgeon retracts with two fingers of the left hand in the abdominal cavity to protect the abdominal viscera and to permit the division of the peritoneum

图 8-4　左手中指和食指插入腹腔，保护内脏，然后用剪刀剪开腹膜

5. Once the peritoneal cavity has been opened and exposed by retractors, exploration of all viscera can be performed, proceeding with the surgery.

（B） Access to abdomen by rectus-splitting incision

1. After skin preparation, surgical field is squared off and draped.

2. The incision has been carried through the skin, the subcutaneous tissue and the anterior rectal sheath at the point about 2 cm from midline. The rectus has been splitted between hemostatic clamps.

3. Using two hemostatic clamps, the posterior rectus sheath and the anterior parietal peritoneum have been grasped (Fig. 8-3). Care should be taken to avoid including the small bowel. The surgeon is about to incise the posterior rectus sheath with scalpel, together with the parietal peritoneum.

Once the abdominal cavity has been opened, the incision is completed using several hemostatic clamps on both edges to apply traction in opposite directions while the peritoneal incision is carried upward and downward using scissors, and the first assistant continues to apply hemostatic clamps to the edges of the peritoneum.

C. Appendectomy

1. Cecum of dog and rabbit is situated in central abdomen (referring to Appendix 1 and 2) and located at the junction between ileum and colon. The appendix is 10 cm long extending from the inferior tip of the cecum in dogs.

The cecum is identified by the large diameter in rabbits and the presence of taenia coli on its surface. First grasp the cecum with non-teethed ring forceps and deliver it to the incision wound. At the earliest opportunity place a Babcock's tissue forceps around the appendix and bring it to the surface. The operative field is isolated with large square packs, the margins of the abdominal incision being covered with protective gauze or an impermeable barrier to guard against contamination.

2. Once the appendix has been delivered, the both sides of visceral peritoneum of mesoappendix are divided close to the appendix by scissors, and the appendicular vessels are clipped, divided and ligated from the tip to the base of the organ. For added security pass a transfixion stitch through the mesentery on each side of the artery forceps.

3. With the appendix held vertically, a purse-string seromuscular suture of 1/0 surgical silk is inserted 1 cm away from the base of the appendix. The appendix is crushed at its base with an artery forceps and the crushed area ligatured with 1/0 surgical silk. The ends of the silk thread are cut short leaving approximately 3 mm from the knot.

4. The appendix is grasped by a straight artery forceps at the level 0.5 cm distal to the ligature and the knot is grasped by another straight artery forceps. The appendix is then divided with a scalpel cutting just under the straight artery forceps. The stump is

cleared with three cotton swabs: dipped in carbolic acid, alcohol of 75 per cent, and normal saline. At this moment, all presumed contaminated items should be put into a basin and removed from operative field including the resected appendix, the straight artery forceps grasping the appendix, the knife, the protective gauze and swabs.

5. The assistant holds the straight artery forceps grasping the knot and invaginating the stump into the cecum where it is retained by tightening and tying the purse-string suture with an adequate force to prevent the suture broken. The site of invagination is examined together with the appendicular mensentery to make sure that hemostasis is secure.

6. After counting the sponges, surgical instruments and needles, the abdominal wall is closed in layers.

D. Closing abdominal wall

1. After completing the intraabdominal procedure, the abdominal cavity should be inspected for bleeding and sponges, needles and surgical instruments counted, and then the abdominal wall is ready to close.

2. To close the incision four artery forceps are placed on the peritoneum which is sutured with a continuous absorbable stitch (for animal experiment, 1/0 surgical silk is used), care being taken not accidentally to pick up a piece of bowel with the needle. Sometimes, a sponge or a straight retractor should be inserted between the anterior parietal peritoneum and the bowels or omentum when initiating the closure to protect bowel from accidental stitch, and taken out from abdomen before the peritoneal closure is completed.

3. Wash the wound with normal saline and approximate the line alba by interrupted or over-and-over suture using 1/0 surgical silk. Wash the wound with normal saline once more, remove the skin protective fenestrated drape or towels, and scrub the incision skin with a single application of alcohol before suture the skin.

4. Massive closure: Closure of all abdominal incisions has been greatly simplified by the realization that all heal by forming a block of fibrous tissue, that disruption is overwhelmingly a mechanical problem and that proper distribution of forces by the use of large bites of relatively heavy non-absorbable material is a virtual guarantee against difficulty.

Sutures should be placed at least 1 cm from the wound edge and less than 1 cm apart. Undue tension should be avoided, and suture length should be 4 times the wound length.

实习八　动物手术(麻醉、静脉切开或穿刺、阑尾切除术)

【目的和要求】

1. 通过动物手术,使学生初步了解阑尾切除术的大致过程。目的是掌握手术基本操作,为今后临床实习打下良好而牢固的基础,而不是要求学会哪种手术。

2. 强化手术中无菌技术的全过程,为以后临床实习作准备。

3. 麻醉者(兼巡回护士),学习动物麻醉之实际操作,静脉切开(穿刺)和输液技术,并熟习台下配合工作。

【实习程序】

1. 学生分成5人一组,按分工规定进行工作。麻醉师提前准备动物,进行麻醉、静脉穿刺和输液,同时做好麻醉记录。手术护士最先洗手,其次为第一助手。

2. 学生要预习本指导,然后按本指导进行阑尾切除术。实习结束后,将狗送回动物房;将手术器械洗净、擦干、上油,打扫手术室。

3. 术后由手术者书写手术记录,逐日观察动物情况并填写术后观察(病程)记录,直至伤口拆线为止。交教研室计分存档。

【实习项目】

一、麻醉和建立静脉通道

1. 狗的术前准备和麻醉　参阅本实习指导概述部分。将麻醉后的狗放于手术台上。

2. 静脉切开术　临床上,静脉切开术常用于抢救危重病人的静脉通道建立,以及需要多条静脉通道的病人。用狗进行实验时,其后肢外侧的大隐静脉是静脉切开的常用部位。

(1) 先取一副2 ml或5 ml注射器和针,抽取等渗盐水或葡萄糖溶液,也可用蝶形输液针。准备好静脉滴注装置,并使装置内充满等渗盐水或葡萄糖溶液。

选择粗细适合的灭菌塑料管一根,将塑料管尖端剪成斜面,但不应太尖。连接注射器,灌满注射液,排净空气泡。

(2) 在狗的后腿外侧、踝关节上方3 cm处有一斜行静脉(图8-1)。在此部位剪毛、用酒精涂擦后很容易找到该静脉。将狗侧卧,用手轻捏踝关节上方,一方面可以制动,另一方面可使该静脉充盈、显现。

(3) 手术部位的皮肤消毒、铺巾后,用1%利多卡因麻醉。如果这条狗已经用了腹腔麻醉,那么该步骤可以省略。

(4) 用15号刀片做切口。皮肤切口的方向可以与该静脉平行、交叉或垂直,切口长2 cm。

(5) 左手持有齿镊提起切口皮肤一侧,右手用蚊式血管钳分离皮下组织,并顺静脉长轴在静脉周围纯性分离,游离出约 1.5 cm 一段静脉。用蚊式血管钳在静脉下方穿出、挑起、引出 2 根丝线(图 8-2),远侧线结扎,但不剪断,留作以后牵引用,近侧线暂不打结。

(6) 用 11 号刀片切开静脉,刀片平放,刺入静脉中部后将刀刃转向上切开静脉。注意不要切断静脉。

(7) 将导管的斜面朝上沿静脉向近心端插入 10 cm(不需要插入过长)。将静脉输液管与静脉导管相连接,开始输液。液体进入静脉通畅时,结扎静脉近心端的丝线固定导管和静脉,线结不宜太紧,以免切割静脉导致导管滑脱。剪短两侧结扎线。

(8) 以酒精消毒切口周围皮肤后,用单纯间断缝合法缝合皮肤切口。利用一根缝线结扎固定塑料管,最后剪短结扎线。导管最好另戳孔引出。

(9) 停止静脉输液拔除塑料管时,先剪去固定塑料管的缝线,再拔除塑料管,加压片刻。

3. 静脉穿刺术　临床上,静脉穿刺术常用于获取血标本或静脉输液。兔的血标本采集和静脉输液常用耳缘静脉穿刺。

(1) 先取一副 2 ml 或 5 ml 注射器和一根不超过 3 cm 长的针,抽取等渗盐水或葡萄糖溶液,也可用蝶形输液针。准备好静脉滴注装置,并让装置内充满等渗盐水或葡萄糖溶液。

(2) 在兔耳后缘选定穿刺之静脉,在此部位将毛发剪短或剃毛(也可不处理),在穿刺前用酒精或碘酒消毒。

如果血管细,穿刺有困难,可以用手指在耳缘静脉处弹几下;在耳根部捏住静脉近心端也可以使静脉充盈;硝酸甘油外用膏也可以使耳缘静脉扩张;成年兔用乙酰丙嗪(1 mg)既可制动,又可扩张血管。

(3) 助手用手压住耳静脉近心侧,使静脉充盈。操作者将针与静脉平行做向心性穿刺。针尖进入静脉腔后,继续向前进入少许。回抽针芯见回血后即可注药。如果没有回血,不要退出针头,应该重新穿刺。初学者往往需要穿刺数次才能成功。用新的锐针头有利于穿刺成功。退出针头时,要在穿刺处加压止血。

虽然有关静脉穿刺的书籍不少,但是,实践是掌握该技术的唯一途径。绳索状静脉、萎瘪静脉和滑动的静脉都可能增加静脉穿刺困难。要达到一针见血的效果往往需要多次尝试。第一针从静脉的远心端开始穿刺,若不成功可以在近侧再次尝试穿刺。

二、剖腹术

对每一个腹部手术来说,都有一个最佳切口选择的问题。Maingot 关于切口选择的三项基本要求是:易达性、可延性和牢固性。然而,决定切口选择的因素很多,诸如:拟手术的器官、外科医生的习惯、对速度的要求、病人的体型、肥胖程度以及既往手术瘢痕等。

一般来讲,直切口(包括正中切口和旁正中切口)能提供很好的易达性和可延性,允许切口向上下延长探查整个腹腔。横切口和斜切口的优点是不容易发生切口裂开。

1. 正中切口开腹术

(1) 手术区按常规消毒,铺无菌巾和剖腹单。

(2) 上腹正中作纵形皮肤切口,长约 10 cm。

① 组织切开要点:皮肤切开时,手术者和第一助手分别以左手尺侧压在切口两侧将切

口两侧皮肤绷紧,术者右手执刀(执餐刀式)(图 2-8),刀片与皮肤垂直,用力适当,要一刀切开皮肤全层,尽量避免多次切割,但不切开白线。切口必须按解剖层次分层切开。

② 止血要点:止血是手术基本操作之一,不仅可减少失血,并且能保持手术野的清晰。皮下组织切开即可进行止血,以纱布压住出血处,用血管钳尖端斜着夹住出血点结扎。由于钳夹对组织有损伤,因此止血钳应该尽可能少夹四周组织。止血钳也可以不结扎,用电凝器逐把电凝止血。止血应分层进行。

③ 结扎要点:出血点都夹住后,即可开始逐个结扎。助手先把血管钳尾端竖起(以便术者将线绕过),随即放低血管钳,使其尖端翘起。待第一个结打好后,在助手松开、移去血管钳的同时,将结继续扎紧,然后打第二个结,打成方结,剪线。剪线时留下的线头要短,若是结扎较大血管的线结,线头可留下较长(约 3 mm)。初学剪线时,最好用左手托住剪刀,使它顺着缝线滑下至线结,再将剪刀侧转 45°剪线。这样就可避免线头留得过长(图 2-39)。

(3)皮肤和皮下组织切开并止血后,再铺一块洞巾,将切口两边分别用 Allis 钳与洞巾固定,保护皮肤(防止皮肤的细菌污染切口)。

然后,切开腹白线,显露腹膜外脂肪及其深面菲薄的腹膜。

(4)术者左手执有齿镊子(或血管钳),第一助手右手执血管钳,两人交替钳夹腹膜。检查、确定没有内脏被钳夹时,用刀切开一小切口(图 8-3)。然后用血管钳夹住腹膜的两侧边缘,将其提起,用剪刀剪开腹膜。剪开腹膜时,可用左手中指和食指插入腹腔,保护内脏(图 8-4)。

(5)打开腹腔后,助手用拉钩牵开,协助暴露,然后即可探查,进行有关手术。

2. 经腹直肌切口开腹术

(1)手术区按常规消毒,铺无菌巾和剖腹单。

(2)经腹直肌切口是距正中线约 2 cm 切开皮肤、皮下组织和腹直肌前鞘,用血管钳纵行分开腹直肌。

(3)用两把血管钳夹住后鞘和壁腹膜(图 8-3)。注意勿夹住腹膜深面的肠管。然后用手术刀将后鞘和腹膜一并切开一小口。

进入腹腔后,助手用血管钳夹住切口两缘作对抗牵引,术者用剪刀分别向上和向下剪开后鞘和腹膜,完成腹壁切开。

三、阑尾切除术

(1)在右中上腹区找寻盲肠(参看附录一)。盲肠位于回、结肠交界处。盲肠的盲端是阑尾,长约 10 cm,容易辨认。先用无齿卵圆钳将盲肠提出切口。然后,用 Babcock 钳夹住阑尾拖至腹腔外,周围以湿纱布或防渗透膜垫好防止污染伤口。

(2)剪开阑尾系膜两侧之腹膜,紧贴阑尾逐渐分离、钳夹切断诸血管,一一予以结扎,直至分离至阑尾根部。必要时,缝合结扎血管更为安全。

(3)将阑尾拎直,在阑尾根部周围的结肠上距阑尾根部 1 cm,以 1 号丝线预置一荷包缝合,缝针只穿透浆肌层,不穿进肠腔。用直血管钳于阑尾根部处轻轻钳夹阑尾,再以 1 号丝线结扎。以蚊式血管钳夹住线结,剪去多余的线。

(4)在结扎线远侧约 0.5 cm 处,用直血管钳钳夹阑尾,在两者之间紧贴血管钳用刀切除阑尾，断端腔内依次以纯石炭酸（或碘酊）、75％酒精和盐水棉签涂擦、消毒。切除之阑尾连同钳夹其上的血管钳、切断时用的手术刀、保护阑尾的湿纱布、棉签，均立即放入一弯盘内，视为有菌污染物，不应再接触或使用。

（5）助手持蚊式血管钳，将盲肠残端向荷包内推入，术者收紧并结扎荷包缝线。收紧及结扎荷包缝线时，用力要适当，逐渐收紧，以防断线。检查阑尾残端和系膜血管处理是否满意。

（6）清点纱布、器械、缝针等无误后，按层关腹。

四、关腹术

（1）腹内手术完毕，检查无出血及纱布、器械等存留腹腔内后，即可关腹。

（2）在腹膜（包括后鞘）上、下两角及两边用弯血管钳钳夹，以可吸收线（动物用1号丝线）从下角开始（亦可从上角开始），连续缝合腹膜和后鞘，必要时腹膜下垫一块纱布或压肠板，避免缝住腹内脏器。缝合接近上角时抽出纱布或压肠板，缝至最后处要注意勿留腹膜间隙。剪短缝线。

（3）以无菌等渗盐水冲洗伤口，以1号丝线缝合腹白线（间断缝合或"8"字形缝合）。再次冲洗伤口。撤去保护皮肤的无菌洞巾，以酒精消毒切口两侧皮肤，然后缝合皮肤。

（4）大块缝合：自从人们认识到伤口愈合是形成整块的纤维瘢痕组织，切口裂开的原因是存在强大的机械力，因此，用粗线做大边距的伤口缝合有利于力的均匀分布，降低切口裂开的可能性。

腹壁缝合的边距至少应该达1 cm，针距应小于1 cm。缝线不宜收得太紧，缝线的长度与伤口的长度应该是4∶1。

Session 9　Hands-on training on animal models （anaesthesia，venous cutdown or venopuncture，and splenectomy）

【Goals & requirements】

The goals and requirements in this session are the same as session 8，except the procedure of splenectomy is different from that of appendectomy.

【Progress schedule】

Progress schedule is the same to the session 8，except the procedure of appendectomy is substituted by splenectomy.

【Topics of this session】

A.　Anesthesia & Venous access

1. Preoperative prep and anesthesia for dogs　Please refer to **Course Overview** of this book.

2. Venous cutdown　Please see Session 8 in this book.

3. Venopuncture　Please see Session 8 in this book.

B.　Laparotomy

Please see Session 8 in this book.

C.　Splenectomy

1. After skin preparation，surgical field is squared off and draped.

2. A 10 cm upper abdominal midline incision is used.

3. Insert a pack over intestine loops allowing retraction inferiorly and to the patient's right，with a broad-bladed Deever's retractor or by the assistant's hand. Expose the gastrosplenic ligament and spleen by drawing the omentum or stomach carefully downwards and to the patient's right.

4. If it is difficult to lift the spleen out of the wound，the superior and inferior attachments can be carefully divided between artery forceps，and ligated using surgical silk.

5. When the inferior pole of the spleen is delivered to the surface，the gastrosplenic

ligament will be found, which is thin and short. The splenic artery is closed to the ligament and identified as it is larger in diameter.

6. The splenic artery and vein should be isolated and ligated in order to obtain "autotransfusion" from the blood trapped in the spleen pulp, especially for patients with splenomegaly. To prevent massive bleeding from accidental suture breaking, the assistant should take care for unlocking the artery forceps slowly, but still bite the vessel in place when the surgeon makes a knot, and then locking the forceps again. Make a second knot (double ligatures) around this vessel before removal of forceps to prevent knot loose or slippage and resultant bleeding. Deal with splenic vessels one by one in the same way, especially for important vessels and upper pole vessel.

7. Divide and ligate gastrolienal ligament between two artery forceps. Remove the resected spleen from the operative field. The proximal end of vessels should be doubly ligated.

8. After inspecting once more for possible bleeding point and foreign bodies in the abdomen and counting the sponges, surgical instruments and needles, the abdominal wall is closed in layers.

D. Closing abdominal wall

Please see Session 8 in this book.

实习九 动物手术（麻醉、静脉切开或穿刺、脾切除术）

【目的和要求】

除脾切除术手术步骤不同于阑尾切除术外，要求与实习八同。

【实习程序】

除脾切除术替代阑尾切除术外，其程序与实习八同。小组人员分工轮换。

【实习项目】

一、麻醉和建立静脉通道

1. 狗的术前准备和麻醉：参阅本书概述。

2. 静脉切开术参阅本书实习八。

3. 静脉穿刺术参阅本书实习八。

二、剖腹术

参阅本书实习八。

三、脾切除术

1. 按常规消毒，铺无菌巾、单。

2. 上腹正中切口长 10 cm 开腹。

3. 先用盐水纱布垫将肠襻挡在腹腔的右下侧。找到胃后，衬着盐水纱布提起大网膜或胃并向右下侧牵拉，即可显露胃脾韧带和脾脏。

4. 如脾的上、下端有韧带牵住，可用两把血管钳夹住，在两钳间切断后，用丝线结扎。

5. 将脾脏下极牵到腹腔外，可看到胃脾韧带菲薄、甚短，其中有较多的血管。脾动脉主干紧贴其旁，较其他血管略粗，容易辨认。

6. 分离出脾动脉和脾静脉。先用两把血管钳夹住脾动脉，在两钳间切断、结扎，进行"自体输血"，这在巨脾病人尤其重要，然后，再处理脾静脉。用丝线结扎近侧脾血管一次（离血管钳稍远）。结扎时稍松开血管钳，结扎后仍夹紧血管钳，在结扎线的远侧再结扎一道，去除血管钳（双重结扎）。按同法处理其余脾血管，尤其应注意脾上极血管的处理，防止结扎线断裂和结扎线脱落大出血。

7．将胃脾韧带内的其他血管依次用两把血管钳钳夹，并在其间切断，取出脾脏。胃侧的血管用丝线双重结扎。

8．检查手术区内没有出血点或异物，清点纱布和器械后，按层缝合腹壁切口。

四、关腹术

参阅本书实习八。

Session 10　Hands-on training on animal models （anaesthesia，venous cutdown or venopuncture，enterectomy and end-to-end anastomosis）

【Goals & requirements】

The goals and requirements in this Session are the same as Session 8，except the procedure of enterectomy with end-to-end anastomosis is different from that of appendectomy.

【Progress schedule】

Progress schedule is the same as the Session 8，except the procedure of appendectomy is substituted by enterectomy with end-to-end anastomosis.

【Topics of this session】

A. Anesthesia & Venous access

1. Preoperative prep and anesthesia for dogs　Please refer to **Course Overview** of this book.

2. Venous cutdown　Please see Session 8 in this book.

3. Venopuncture　Please see Session 8 in this book.

B. Laparotomy

Please see Session 8 in this book.

C. Small bowel resection and end-to-end reconstruction

1. After skin preparation，surgical field is squared off and draped.

2. A 10-cm upper abdominal midline incision is used.

3. A segment of jejunum is selected to be resected. A resection length of 5～10 cm is recommended. Important factor which determines the choice of a particular segment of jejunum is the anatomy of the mesenteric vascular arcades to ensure that the vasculature of the remaining small bowel is not undercut during division of the mesentery.

4. After the surgeon has decided upon the extent and lines of resection of the small

intestine, both sides of viscera peritoneum of related mesentery is divided with scissors in a wedge fashion and the blood vessels irrigating the intestine corresponding to the section to be resected are serially clamped and divided between artery forceps, and complete hemostasis is secured by means of suture ligatures of fine silk (Fig. 10-1).

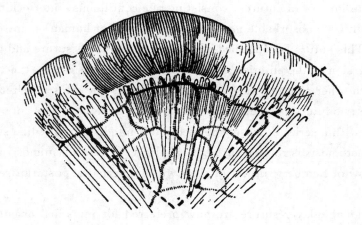

Fig. 10-1   The related mesentery is divided in a wedge fashion
图 10-1   楔性离断肠系膜

5. Either end of the small bowel segment to be cut is placed a Kocher clamp. Two non-crushing intestinal clamps are then applied 3~5 cm away from each Kocher clamp, respectively. The surgical field is isolated with large square packs, the margins of the abdominal incision being covered with protective gauze or an impermeable barrier to guard against contamination. The gut is divided close to the outside of Kocher clamp with a cautery or knife (Fig. 10-2), the segment containing the devascularized bowel removed, and any intestinal contents are removed by suction or by mopping with small swabs.

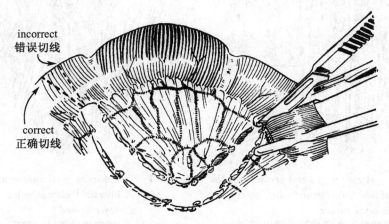

Fig. 10-2   The gut is cut close to the outside of Kocher clamp
图 10-2   在 Kocher 钳外侧紧贴该钳断离肠襻

6. The continuity of the small bowel is restored by means of an end-to-end anastomo-

sis which is carried out in two layers using 1/0 surgical silk thread sutures.

7. The proximal and distal segments to be united are held together, and two seromuscular stay sutures (1/0 silk) were placed through both segments on the mesenteric and antimesenteric borders, respectively, to stabilize the position of the segments relative to each other. The posterior row of sutures, consisting of a continuous, interlocking (lock-stitch) strand of 1/0 silk (000 absorbable material is the choice for human) is introduced through all the layers. This suture is continued anteriorly as a Connell suture and produces a near water-tight inversion of the anterior margins of the intestine. Then, the two ends of the thread meet each other and are tied with the knot inside the intestinal lumen (Fig. 3-8, Fig. 3-9). The two intestinal clamps are unlocked and removed. The anterior surfaces are joined together with a series of closely applied interrupted sutures of fine silk (Fig. 3-6). At last, the anastomosis is rotated through 180 degrees. The anastomosis is completed by introducing a row of Lembert sutures of silk, which inverts the posterior seromuscular suture line.

Interrupted single-layer suture are now preferred for intestinal anastomoses. A 1/0 (round bodied needle) silk suture is passed through all layer, 5 mm from the cut edge and 5～6 mm apart, through the proximal and distal bowel (inside-out-out-inside for posterior wall with knots tied inside the intestinal lumen and out-in-in-out for anterior wall with knots tied outside) and tied (Fig. 10-3, Fig. 10-4). A mid-point marking suture aids accurate tissue apposition.

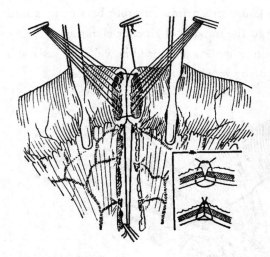 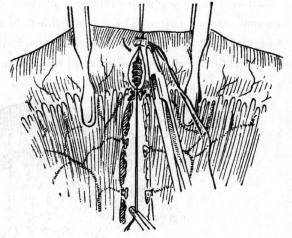

Fig. 10-3　The posterior wall anastomosis with the aid of intestinal clamps using interrupted single-layer suture

Fig. 10-4　The anterior wall anastomosis with the aid of intestinal clamps using interrupted single-layer suture

图 10-3　在肠钳辅助下进行后壁一层间断缝合　　　图 10-4　在肠钳辅助下进行前壁一层间断缝合

8. Check all the sutures and test the patency of the stroma with thumb and index finger (Fig. 3-7).

9. The defect in the mesentery is closed by approximating the peritoneal edges with interrupted silk sutures (Fig. 10-5).

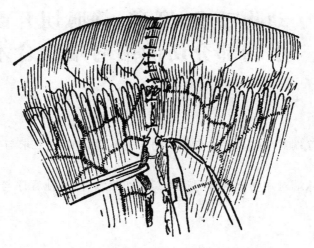

Fig. 10-5   Close the defect of the mesentery
图 10-5   间断缝合肠系膜孔

10. Inspect once more for possible bleeding point take gauze and pad out from the abdomen and count. Close the abdominal wall.

D. Closing abdominal wall

Please see Session 8 in this book.

实习十 动物手术(麻醉、静脉切开或穿刺、小肠部分切除端对端吻合术)

【目的和要求】

除小肠部分切除端对端吻合手术步骤不同于阑尾切除术外,要求与实习八同。

【实习程序】

除小肠部分切除端对端吻合术步骤替代阑尾切除术外,其他程序与实习八同。小组人员分工轮换。

【实习项目】

一、麻醉和建立静脉通道

1. 狗的术前准备和麻醉:参阅本书概述。

2. 静脉切开术参阅本书实习八。

3. 静脉穿刺术参阅本书实习八。

二、剖腹术

参阅本书实习八。

三、小肠部分切除端对端吻合术

1. 按常规消毒,铺无菌巾、单。

2. 上腹部正中切口长 10 cm 进腹。

3. 选择一段拟切除的肠管,建议切除肠管 5～10 cm。此时,要注意肠系膜的血管弓解剖,要求在肠切除后,保留肠管的血供良好。

4. 在小肠的切除范围和切断线确定后,用剪刀楔形剪开两侧系膜的腹膜层,分出相应的血管弓,切断、结扎(图 10-1)。

5. 在拟切除肠段的两端各上一把 Kocher 钳,再在 Kocher 钳外侧 3～5 cm 处各上一把肠钳。铺大纱垫或保护膜防止手术野被肠内容物溢出污染。用电刀或手术刀紧贴 Kocher 钳切断肠管(图 10-2),移去切除的肠段,残端肠腔的内容物用吸引器吸去或用棉球擦去。

6. 本实验中,消化道连续性的重建方式是两层端端吻合。

7. 将肠襻的两断端平行放好,分别在肠的系膜缘和对系膜缘各做一针浆肌层缝合用于牵引。先用 1/0 丝线(在病人一般用 000 可吸收缝线)做后壁全层连续锁边缝合,继续用这根线做前壁全层连续 Connell 缝合，使吻合口内翻（图 3-8，图 3-9）。全层缝合的两个线头相遇后，相互打结，线结打在肠腔内。松开并移去两把肠钳。用间断 Lembert 缝合法缝合前壁浆肌层。然后将肠襻翻转 180°，用间断 Lembert 缝合法完成后壁浆肌层的缝合（图 3-6）。

如今，临床上一般用一层间断缝合进行肠吻合。可以用 1/0 丝线圆针在肠的两端之间做端端全层吻合，边距 5 mm，针距 5～6 mm，后壁吻合的进针是内—外—外—内，前壁吻合的进针是外—内—内—外（图 10-3，图 10-4）。每次从中间进针有助于组织的对合。

8. 检查吻合口是否满意，并用拇指和食指试探吻合口的大小（图 3-7）。

9. 小肠系膜孔用丝线间断缝合关闭（图 10-5）。

10. 检查腹内无出血或异物，取出腹内纱布，点数。按层缝合腹壁切口。

四、关腹术

参阅本书实习八。

Session 11　Hands-on training on animal models（anaesthesia，venous cutdown or venopuncture，partial gastrectomy and gastrojejunal anastomosis）

【Goals & requirements】
Please see Session 10 in this book.

【Progress schedule】
Please see Session 10 in this book.

【Topics of this session】
Please see Session 10 in this book.

实习十一 动物手术（麻醉、静脉切开或穿刺、胃部分切除、胃空肠吻合术）

【目的和要求】

参见实习十。

【实习程序】

参见实习十。

【实习项目】

参见实习十。

Session 12　Hands-on training on animal models （anaesthesia，venous cutdown or venopuncture，partial gastrectomy and gastrojejunal anastomosis）

【Goals & requirements】

The goals and requirements in this session are the same as Session 8，except the procedure of partial gastrectomy and gastrojejunal anastomosis is different from that of appendectomy.

【Progress schedule】

Progress schedule is the same as Session 8，except for the procedure of partial gastrectomy and gastrojejunal anastomosis.

【Topics of this session】

A. Anesthesia & Venous access

1. Preoperative prep and anesthesia for dogs　Please refer to **Course Overview** of this book.

2. Venous cutdown　Please see Session 8 in this book.

3. Venopuncture　Please see Session 8 in this book.

B. Laparotomy

Please see Session 8 in this book.

C. Partial gastrectomy and gastrojejunal anastomosis

1. After skin preparation，surgical field is squared off and draped.

2. A mid-line epigastric incision is commonly used.

3. The division of the gastrocolic omentum begins in the avascular area to the left，below the short gastric vessels，and inside the gastro-epiploic arch (Fig. 12-1). Division is easiest outside the arcade but in obese patients the risk of postoperative fat necrosis is increased.

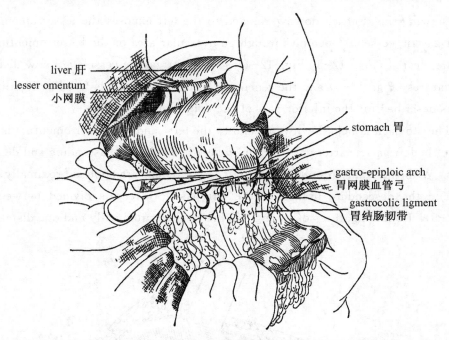

liver 肝
lesser omentum
小网膜
stomach 胃
gastro-epiploic arch
胃网膜血管弓
gastrocolic ligment
胃结肠韧带

Fig. 12-1 Separation of the gastrocolic omentum inside the gastro-epiploic arch
图 12-1 在胃网膜血管弓内侧游离胃的大弯侧

4. The stomach is turned upwards and medially to allow division of adhesions between the posterior wall and the pancreas and proceed to the right exposes the right gastro-epiploic vessels which should be divided close to and below the pylorus. Sharp dissection may occasionally be required as the dissection proceeds to the right to expose the posterior wall of the duodenum (Fig. 12-2). Here fine forceps are required to deal with vessels until the posterior duodenal wall is cleared.

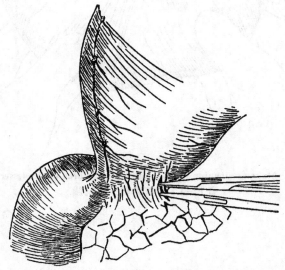

Fig. 12-2 Turn the stomach upwards and separate the posterior wall of the pylorus and the duodenum
图 12-2 上翻胃,在胃窦和十二指肠与胰腺之间分离

5. Drawing the stomach downwards and to the left exposes the lesser omentum and the right gastric vessels. Opening through an avascular area of the lesser omentum these vessels are cleared (Fig. 12-3, Fig. 12-4). The right gastric vessels are now divided between ligatures (Fig. 12-4) and the remainder of the duodenum is freed by ligating small vessels as described for the inferior part of the duodenum.

6. The stomach is held downwards and to the left, and the lesser omentum is divided to expose the left gastric artery at the point where it divides into ascending and descending branches. With the stomach pulled to the left, two forceps are applied proximally and one distally and the descending branch of the left gastric artery is divided between them (Fig. 12-5). Double ligatures of strong silk are applied proximally and one distally.

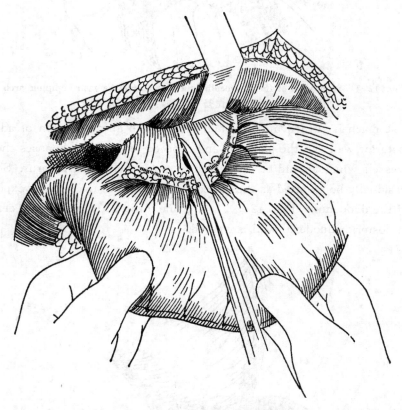

Fig. 12-3 Make an opening through an avascular area of the lesser omentum
图 12-3 用剪刀剪开小网膜

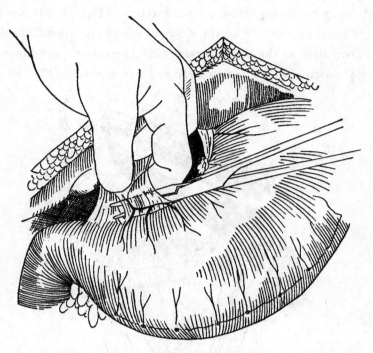

Fig. 12-4   Divide the right gastric vessels between ligatures or clamps
图 12-4   分离、结扎胃右血管

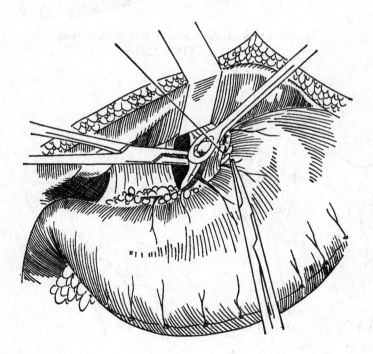

Fig. 12-5   Divide the left gastric artery between clamps
图 12-5   分离、结扎胃左血管

7. The duodenum is divided between Kocher clamps (Fig. 12-6), and a gauze swab is used to cover the proximal part. With the Kocher clamp in position Connell suture of silk may be used, drawn tight as the clamp is removed. Thereafter a continuous seromuscular running sutures are used with the same thread as Connell suture (Fig. 12-7).

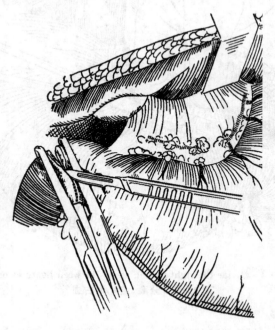

Fig. 12-6　Divide duodenum between Kocher clamps
图 12-6　切断十二指肠

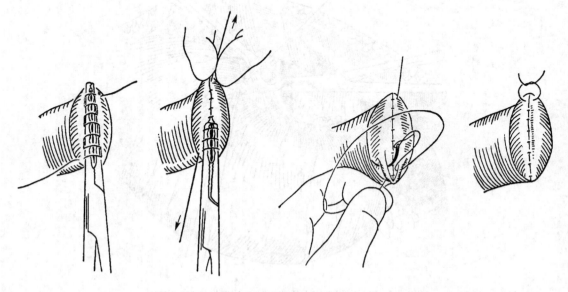

Fig. 12-7　Closure of the duodenal stump
图 12-7　十二指肠残端的缝合

The stomach is now cleared and the site for anastomosis selected (Fig. 12 – 8, Fig. 12–9). In general a 1/2 gastrectomy is carried out but this may be difficult to judge.

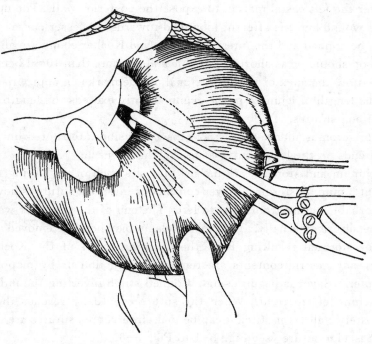

Fig. 12–8　The cutting line for distal gastrectomy

图 12－8　远端胃切除术的切断线

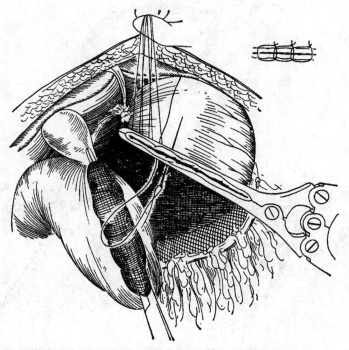

Fig. 12–9　Divide the stomach between clamps

图 12－9　切断胃

8. A Kocher clamp is placed across the stomach at the level selected. Stomach should be preserved as much as possible to make the anastomosis easy and safe. The stomach is then pulled over the left costal margin to expose the posterior wall. The upper jejunum is pulled into the wound and the afferent loop held towards the lesser curve，when a intestinal clamp may be applied and the intestinal clamp and Kocher clamp are aligned together. The afferent loop should be as short as possible and no more than 10～12 cm from the duodenojejunal flexure；the apex of the first jejunal arcade marks an appropriate length. It is preferable if the length of jejunum in the clamp slightly exceeds the length of stomach for easy control of end sutures.

A posterior seromuscular suture is now inserted using interrupted fine silk beginning to the left and ends on the lesser curve aspect of the stomach.

9. The jejunum and stomach are incised opposite each other leaving a seromuscular margin of about 3 mm. Posterior all-layer continuous interlock suture is now applied using a separate absorbable suture from right to left. The end of the posterior wall is completed by bringing the suture externally. The Kocher clamp may now be removed and the devitalized margins of stomach resulting from the crushing effect of the Kocher clamps are trimmed away，any gastric contents are removed by suction or by mopping with small swabs. The anterior layer is begun using a Connell stitch inverting the mucosa as the suture proceeds from left to right. When the suture eventually reaches the initial suture starting the posterior all-layer stitch it can be tied. Interrupted sutures are then applied for anterior seromuscular suture （see Fig. 3-1 to Fig. 3-6）.

Interrupted single-layer suture are now preferred for gastrojejunal anastomosis （Fig. 12-10）.

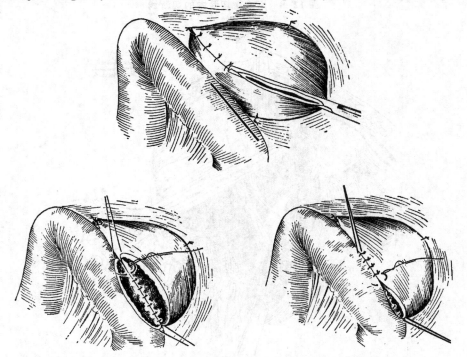

Fig. 12-10 Gastrojejunal anastomosis using interrupted single-layer suture
图 12-10 胃空肠一层间断缝合

10. Final inspection: Before closing the abdomen a general inspection for bleeding is carried out with particular reference to the spleen, vascular pedicles and omentum.

D. Closing abdominal wall

Please see Session 8 in this book.

实习十二 动物手术（麻醉、静脉切开或穿刺、胃部分切除、胃空肠吻合术）

【目的和要求】

除胃部分切除、胃空肠吻合术手术的步骤不同于阑尾切除术外，要求与实习八同。

【实习程序】

除手术操作步骤不同于阑尾切除术外，其余与实习八同。小组人员分工轮换。

【实习项目】

一、麻醉和建立静脉通道

1. 狗的术前准备和麻醉：参阅本书概述。
2. 静脉切开术参阅本书实习八。
3. 静脉穿刺术参阅本书实习八。

二、剖腹术

参阅本书实习八。

三、胃部分切除、胃空肠吻合术

1. 按常规消毒，铺无菌巾、单。
2. 上腹部正中切口开腹。
3. 在胃网膜血管弓内侧无血管区向左侧分离胃网膜血管弓至胃短血管处（图 12-1）。当然，在胃网膜血管弓外分离该血管弓更方便，但是在肥胖人容易发生大网膜坏死。
4. 用手捏住胃大弯，将胃提至切口，向右游离大网膜，在幽门下切断结扎胃网膜右血管。上翻胃，可见胃窦与胰腺之间有腹膜相连，在无血管区剪开腹膜，使胃窦与胰腺之间得以分离（图 12-2）。向右分离胃网膜血管弓，在幽门下将其切断结扎。
5. 向下牵拉胃，显露小网膜和胃右血管，用剪刀剪开小网膜（图 12-3）。分离、结扎胃右血管（图 12-4）。然后，用蚊式血管钳处理十二指肠后的小血管，游离十二指肠球部。
6. 向左下牵引胃，分离小网膜，显露胃左动脉及其升支和降支的交会点。在胃左动脉降支的近侧上两把血管钳，远侧上一把血管钳，在其间剪断胃左动脉降支（图 12-5）。近侧断端双重结扎，远侧断端单扎。
7. 用两把 Kocher 钳夹住十二指肠球部，用手术刀在其间切断十二指肠（图 12-6），近

148

断端用纱布包裹。十二指肠残端的 Kocher 钳不松开，用 Connell 缝合法缝闭十二指肠残端，边移去 Kocher 钳，边收紧缝线。然后，继续用这根线做连续浆肌层缝合加强（图 12-7）。

此时，胃的远端已经全部游离，拟定胃的切除线（图 12-8，图 12-9）。通常切除 1/2 胃即可，不要切除过多。

8. 用 Kocher 钳按预订切除线钳夹胃，尽可能多留胃组织，便于吻合。将胃翻至左肋弓上方，显露胃后壁。将近端空肠提至切口，使输入襻对胃小弯，用肠钳夹住拟吻合的空肠襻。肠钳和 Kocher 钳平行放置。要求输入襻距十二指肠空肠曲不超过 10～12 cm，空肠的第一个血管弓可以作为标志。肠钳钳夹空肠时，空肠的长度应该略长于胃，以便于两端的吻合操作。

然后，用细丝线做后壁浆肌层间断缝合，从大弯缝向小弯侧。

9. 距后壁浆肌层缝线 3 mm 切开空肠和胃。从小弯侧开始用可吸收线做胃后壁全层毯边连续缝合，吻合线缝至大弯侧时，用刀紧贴 Kocher 钳切去钳夹的胃组织，移去 Kocher 钳，吸去或擦去胃内容物。将缝针穿至浆膜外，转向前壁，行前壁全层单纯连续吻合或 Connell 缝合，从大弯侧向小弯侧。两线头相互打结，线结打在胃腔内。移去 Kocher 钳和肠钳。最后行前壁浆肌层间断缝合（图 3-1～图 3-6）。

一层间断缝合法也可用于胃空肠吻合（图 12-10）。

10. 关腹前常规检查腹内无出血，特别要注意脾脏、血管蒂结扎处和网膜。

四、关腹术

参阅实习八。

Appendix 1　The choice of the incision
for abdominal surgery in dogs

The anatomy of dog is different from human. It is wise to study the related anatomy of dog before performing abdominal surgery in dog. A suitable incision gives good access and excellent exposure to special organ, and a wrong incision will make the operation hard.

The length of the abdomen is long, the subcostal angle is narrow and the level of umbilicus is higher in dogs. Liver, gallbladder and stomach are located in upper part of the abdominal cavity protected by rib cage and are hardly exposed. Cecum and spleen are freely mobile and can be easily accessed.

A. Location of abdominal viscera in dogs

For purpose of description, the abdomen is customarily divided into quadrants that intersect at umbilicus (Fig. 1).

1. The right upper quadrant: liver, pylorus (at the level of xiphoid process), gall bladder (at the level of xiphoid process), common bile duct, duodenum and a part of pancreas, right adrenal gland, and right kidney or upper pole of right kidney.

2. The left upper quadrant: stomach (the lower point of the greater curvature at the level of umbilicus and lesser curvature at the level of xiphoid process), the left part of liver, the upper pole of spleen, left adrenal gland, left kidney or upper pole of left kidney, and a part of pancreas.

3. The left lower quadrant: small bowel, left kidney or lower pole of left kidney, the lower pole of spleen or most part of the spleen, left part of urinary bladder, colon and rectum.

4. The right lower quadrant: small bowel, lower pole of right kidney (may or may not present), colon and right part of urinary bladder.

Cecum joins the colon at the level and a little bit right to the umbilicus. There are uterus, ovaries and fallopian tube in the lower quadrants of female dogs.

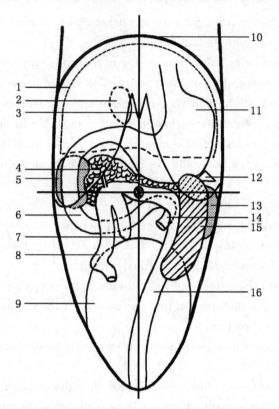

Fig. 1   Location of abdominal viscera for dogs（small bowel is resected）

1. liver；2. gall bladder；3. xiphoid process；4. pancreas；5. right kidney；6. duodenum；7. cecum；8. terminal ileum；9. distended urinary bladder；10. top part of diaphragm；11. stomach；12. left adrenal gland；13. left kidney；14. duodenojejunal flexure；15. spleen；16. rectum.

图 1   狗腹腔脏器部位投影图（小肠已切除）

1.肝；2.胆囊；3.剑突；4.胰腺；5.右肾；6.十二指肠；7.盲肠；8.回肠末端；9.膨胀的膀胱；10.膈肌顶部；11.胃；12.左肾上腺；13.左肾；14.十二指肠空肠曲；15.脾；16.直肠。

B. Choice of incision and key points for surgery

1. A vertical periumbilical incision, right paramedian or right midrectus (rectus-splitting), may be used for cecectomy or appendectomy. Periumbilical incision, left paramedian or left midrectus (rectus-splitting), may be used for splenectomy and enterectomy. If cecectomy and splenectomy will be done simultaneously, either median or right paramedian incision can be chosen as both of appendix and spleen are very mobile.

2. Lower abdominal incision, which is a common mistake made by learners, is not appreciated because of the distended urinary bladder which can obscure exposure.

3. Duodenum is very short in dog and includes just the area where the pancreas and bile ducts empty into the intestines. Duodenal mesentery is wide and contains the pancreas which is mobile tissue and attach the pylorus.

4. Except the splenic pedicle, greater omentum in dog is very thin and loaded with lit-

tle fat. The omentum hangs from the greater curvature of stomach as an apron over bowels but is not attached to colon as human.

5. Similar to human being, the colon in dog is also consisting of ascending, transverse and descending, but the ascending colon is short. Colon becomes rectum as it goes distally and there are no sigmoid colon, and no taeniae coli and appendices epiploicae on colon in dogs. Whole colon has it short mesentery so colon is movable in dogs. Cecum meets the colon at the junction of the terminal ileum and colon. Mesocecum is short, in which there is blood vessels. These vessels should be isolated and divided during the procedure of cecectomy.

6. There are three ways to find the cecum:

(1) Once the abdominal cavity is entered, displace omentum upward to find the cecum right to the umbilicus at umbilical plane. The cecum is grey-blue without contents and turns to pink as small intestine when it is filled with gas.

(2) Look for colon (the outer longitudinal muscle layer can be identified) at umbilical plane, and follow it in one direction to find the cecum. If the cecum can not be found, try to drag it in an opposite direction.

(3) Drag the omentum downward and you will find the ileocecal junction and cecum. Deliver it to the wound.

7. The way to find spleen: The spleen is closed to the incision if epigastric or left periumbilical vertical incision is made. If the incision is made on the right, the spleen, except the upper pole of the spleen which is fixed, can be delivered into the wound by gently dragging the greater omentum.

8. The ligamentum teres runs along the inferior edge of the falciform ligament from the umbilicus to the umbilical fissure of liver at the middle of epigastrium and protrudes to the abdominal cavity as if an omentum. Epigastric midline incision is carried out in this plane where the extraperitoneal fat is abundant, and vascular, and small vessels here need to be coagulated with diathermy.

9. The anterior pleural reflection is at the level of the middle of xiphoid. The epigastric incision can not be extended to this level in order to avoid entering the pleura and resultant open pneumothorax.

10. A distended urinary bladder may reach at the level of upper third and lower two thirds of the length of lower abdomen, and even to the level of umbilicus, so lower abdominal incision is avoided.

附录一　狗的腹部解剖和手术切口选择

狗的解剖不同于人,在进行狗腹部手术时,必须了解狗的腹腔解剖,根据狗腹腔脏器位置,选用适当切口,才能得到满意的显露,否则,必将增加手术的困难。

狗腹部较长,肋间角较小,脐的位置较高。肝脏、胆囊和胃位于上腹部,显露较困难。盲肠、脾位于中腹部,显露较容易。

一、狗腹腔脏器位置

如以一正中垂直线和一条通过脐之水平线将狗腹部分为四个象限,则腹腔脏器位置分布如下(图1):

1. 右上象限:肝,胃幽门部(平剑突),胆囊(平剑突),胆总管,十二指肠和胰腺的一部分,右肾上腺,右肾(或仅右肾上极)。

2. 左上象限:胃(下缘平脐、小弯平剑突),肝脏之左侧部分,脾脏上极,左肾上腺,左肾上极(有时在脐水平线以下),胰腺的一部分。

3. 左下象限:小肠,左肾(或其下极),脾脏之下极(或大部分),膀胱之左半,结肠,直肠。

4. 右下象限:小肠,右肾下极(或无),结肠,膀胱之右半。

此外,盲肠多位于脐水平线、脐右侧附近;雌狗下腹部有子宫、卵巢和输卵管。

二、手术切口选择及注意点

1. 盲肠(阑尾)切除术可选用正中绕脐、右旁正中或右经腹直肌切口;脾切除术可选用正中绕脐、左旁正中或左经腹直肌切口。切口应以脐平面为中点,因盲肠和脾脏均在此平面,且可上下兼顾。正中绕脐和右旁正中切口进行小肠部分切除术亦很方便。狗的盲肠和脾脏游离度较大,如同时进行盲肠切除术和脾切除术,切口位于任何一侧均可显露。

2. 手术切口不能过低,否则膨胀的膀胱往往占据切口的一部分或大部分,造成手术显露困难。手术切口过低,是学生在手术中常犯错误之一。

3. 十二指肠有较宽的肠系膜,其2、3段系膜中包藏着游动的胰腺。

4. 除脾蒂附近外,大网膜上脂肪一般不多。大网膜不与横结肠相连,由胃大弯向下掩盖腹部。

5. 结肠亦分升、横、降等部,升结肠甚短,降结肠下降后即为直肠相续,无明显的乙状结肠。全部结肠皆有肠系膜,但均较短,无结肠带和脂肪垂。盲肠位于回肠与升结肠相交之角内并卧向回肠末端,盲肠系膜甚短,其内的血管亦横卧于盲肠与回肠末端之间。在盲肠切除分离系膜血管时,可分开其两侧之腹膜,细心分离其间之血管。

6．寻找盲肠之方法有以下三种：

（1）开腹后，将大网膜上推，于脐水平脐的右侧直接寻找盲肠。未充盈的盲肠，略显淡蓝色；当推挤充气后，则色泽与小肠相似。

（2）于脐平面先寻找结肠（外观为纵行纤维），将其向一个方向牵拉，如未能找到，再向相反方向牵拉，即能找到盲肠。

（3）将大网膜提起后尽量向下方牵拉，位于回肠和结肠交角处的盲肠，可被牵向腹腔浅部，在切口中被显露。

7．寻找脾脏的方法：如系左中、上腹切口，开腹后即可见到脾脏；如系右侧切口，将大网膜提起后向右下牵拉，即可将脾脏牵出切口，但脾脏的上极较固定，难以显露。

8．上腹正中线相当于肝圆韧带部分，在腹膜外有较多量脂肪，以致使腹膜向腹腔内突出，状似网膜。上腹正中切口需经过此区，其中有较多血管（多为静脉），术中必须妥加处理。

9．胸膜反折线位于剑突中部的平面，故上腹手术切口的上限不可超过此平面，否则即可切开胸膜，导致开放性气胸。

10．术前未排尿者，膨胀之膀胱可上升至下腹上中 1/3 交界处，甚至达脐平面。一般应避免选用下腹部切口。

Appendix 2   The choice of the incision for abdominal surgery in rabbits

The anatomy of rabbit is different from human. It is wise to study the related anatomy of rabbit before performing abdominal surgery in rabbit. A well-placed incision should bring the surgeon immediately onto the special organ, and a wrong incision will make the operation hard.

The rabbit is herbivorous mammal that has a larger stomach than the cat to store large amounts of grasses. It has a longer small intestine and a very long "sac-like" cecum for hindgut fermentation of grasses. As a result, the length of the abdomen is long, the subcostal angle is narrow and the level of umbilicus is higher in rabbits. Liver, gall bladder and stomach are located in upper part of the abdomen protected by rib cage and are hardly exposed. Cecum and spleen are freely mobile and can be easily accessed.

A. Location of abdominal viscera in rabbits

For purposes of description, the abdomen is customarily divided into quadrants that intersect at umbilicus (Fig. 1).

1. The right upper quadrant: liver, pylorus (at the level of xiphoid process), gall bladder (at the level of xiphoid process), common bile duct, duodenum and a part of pancreas, right adrenal gland, right kidney or upper pole of right kidney, and cecum.

2. The left upper quadrant: stomach (the lower point of the greater curvature at the level of umbilicus and lesser curvature at the level of xiphoid process), the left part of liver, the upper pole of spleen, left adrenal gland, left kidney or upper pole of left kidney, a part of pancreas, and cecum.

3. The left lower quadrant: small bowel, left kidney or lower pole of left kidney, the lower pole of spleen or most part of the spleen, left part of urinary bladder, cecum, appendix, colon and rectum.

4. The right lower quadrant: small bowel, lower pole of right kidney (may or may not present), colon and right part of urinary bladder.

Cecum joins the colon at the level and a little bit right to the umbilicus. There are uterus, ovaries and salpinx in the lower quadrants for female rabbits.

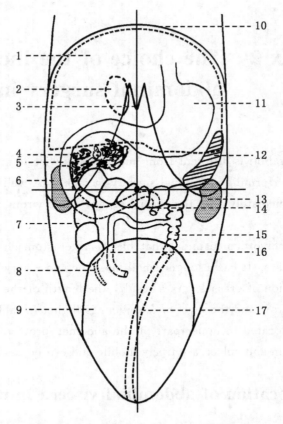

Fig. 1　Location of abdominal viscera for rabbits（small bowel is resected）
1. liver；2. gall bladder；3. xiphoid process；4. pancreas；5. duodenum；6. right kidney；7. cecum；8. appendix；9. distended urinary bladder；10. top part of diaphragm；11. stomach；12. spleen；13. left kidney；14. duodenojejunal flexure；15. colon；16. distal part of ileum；17. rectum.

图 1　兔腹腔脏器部位投影图（小肠已切除）
1. 肝；2. 胆囊；3. 剑突；4. 胰腺；5. 十二指肠；6. 右肾；7. 盲肠；8. 阑尾；9. 膨胀的膀胱；10. 膈肌顶部；11. 胃；12. 脾脏；13. 左肾；14. 十二指肠空肠曲；15. 结肠；16. 回肠末端；17. 直肠。

B. Choice of incision and key points for surgery

1. Vertical periumbilical incisions，median or right paramedian，may be used for appendectomy. Epigastric median incision is excellent for partial gastrectomy. If appendectomy and splenectomy will be done simultaneously，either median or right paramedian incision can be chosen as both of appendix and spleen are very mobile.

2. Lower abdominal incision，which is a common mistake made by learners，is not appreciated because of the distended urinary bladder which can obscure exposure.

3. Duodenum is very short in rabbit and includes just the area where the pancreas and bile ducts empty into the intestines. Duodenal mesentery is wide and contains the pancreas which is mobile tissue and attach the pylorus.

4. Except the splenic pedicle, greater omentum in rabbit is very thin and loaded with little fat. The omentum hangs from the greater curvature of stomach as an apron over bowels but not adherent to colon as in human.

5. The rabbit is herbivorous mammal that has a very long (about 40 cm in length) and large (4 cm in diameter) cecum which shows royal blue, occupies most space in the abdomen and involves all four quadrants. The cecum ends with an appendix which is a conical diverticulum. The appendix in adult rabbit averages 10 cm in length and 1.5 cm in diameter at the base and 1.0 cm in diameter at the tip. The appendiceal artery is a branch of the ileocolic artery (Fig. 2). The ileocolic artery should not be compromised during the procedure of appendectomy. The appendix can be found by following the cecum with large diameter in rabbits.

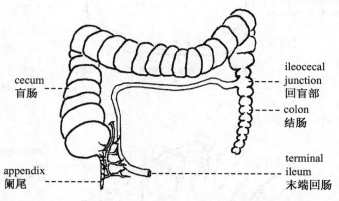

cecum
盲肠

ileocecal
junction
回盲部

colon
结肠

terminal
ileum
末端回肠

appendix
阑尾

Fig. 2   The anatomy of cecum, ileum and appendix, and their blood supplies in rabbit cecum, appendix, ileocecal junction, colon, terminal ileum

图 2   兔的回肠、盲肠与结肠及阑尾血供的解剖示意图

6. The proximal end of cecum meets the colon at the junction of the terminal ileum and colon. Colon is pink and averages 1.5~2.0 cm; as colon proceeds distally, the lumen narrows, and contents become more solid and oval. Different from human being, there are no ascending and transverse colon, and no taeniae coli and appendices epiploicae on colon in rabbits, but whole colon has its short mesentery so colon is movable in rabbits. Colon becomes rectum as it runs distally.

7. The way to find spleen: The spleen is closed to the incision if epigastric or left periumbilical vertical incision is made. If the incision is made on the right, the spleen, except the upper pole of the spleen which is fixed, can be delivered into the wound by gently dragging the greater omentum.

8. The blood supply to the stomach in rabbits is similar to human, but the right gastric artery distributes the stomach at angular incisure, which should be divided when gastrectomy is carried out (Fig. 3, Fig. 4).

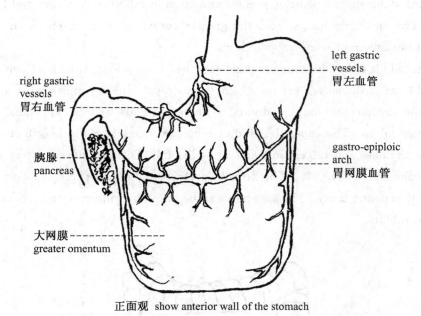

正面观 show anterior wall of the stomach

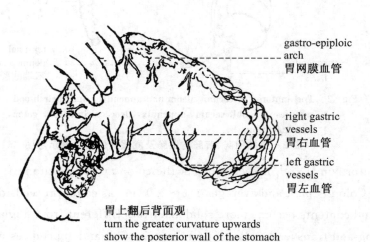

胃上翻后背面观
turn the greater curvature upwards
show the posterior wall of the stomach

Fig. 3   The blood supply to the stomach in rabbits
图3   兔的胃血供示意图

9. The anterior pleural reflection is at the level of the middle of xiphoid. The epigastric incision can not be extended to this level in order to avoid entering the pleura and resultant open pneumothorax.

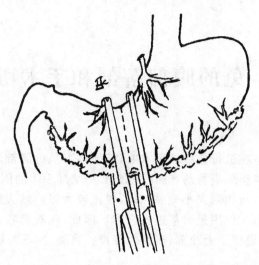

**Fig. 4   The proposed line of section for distal gastrectomy
and right gastric artery division**
图 4   远端胃切除时需要切断胃右血管

10. A distended urinary bladder may reach at the level of upper third and lower two thirds of the length of lower abdomen, and even to the level of umbilicus, so lower abdominal incision is avoided.

附录二　兔的腹部解剖和手术切口选择

兔的解剖不同于人。在进行兔腹部手术前,必须学习兔的腹部解剖。根据兔腹腔脏器位置,选用适当切口,才能得到满意的显露,否则,必将增加手术的困难。

兔是食草动物,因此,与相同大小的猫相比,胃比较大以容纳大量的草。兔的小肠也比较长,盲肠很长呈"囊状",其作用是对草进行发酵。因此,兔腹部较长,肋间角较小,脐位于较高平面。肝脏、胆囊和胃位于上腹部,显露较困难。盲肠、脾较游离,显露较容易。

一、兔腹腔脏器位置

如以一正中垂直线和一条通过脐之水平线将兔腹部分为四个象限,则腹腔脏器位置分布如下(图 1):

1. 右上象限:肝,胃幽门部(平剑突),胆囊(平剑突),胆总管,十二指肠和胰腺的一部分,右肾上腺,右肾(或仅右肾上极)和盲肠。

2. 左上象限:胃(下缘平脐、小弯平剑突),肝脏之左侧部分,脾脏上极,左肾上腺,左肾上极(有时在脐平线以下),胰腺的一部分和盲肠。

3. 左下象限:小肠,左肾(或其下极),脾脏之下极(或大部分),膀胱之左半,盲肠,阑尾,结肠,直肠。

4. 右下象限:小肠,右肾下极(或无),盲肠,膀胱之右半。

此外,盲肠结肠交界多位于脐平线、脐右侧附近;雌兔下腹部有子宫、卵巢和输卵管。

二、手术切口选择及手术注意点

1. 阑尾切除术可选用右旁正中或中腹部正中切口;脾切除术可选用上腹正中切口。上腹正中切口进行胃部分切除术亦很方便。兔的阑尾和脾脏游离度较大,如同时进行阑尾切除术和脾切除术,切口位于任何一侧均可显露。

2. 手术切口不能过低,否则膨胀的膀胱往往占据切口的一部分或大部分,造成手术显露困难。手术切口过低,是学生在手术中常犯错误之一。

3. 十二指肠有较宽的肠系膜,其 2、3 段系膜中包藏着游动的胰腺,胰腺与胃窦部紧密相连。

4. 除脾蒂附近外,大网膜菲薄,无脂肪,大网膜不与横结肠相连,由胃大弯下垂,掩盖小肠。

5. 兔为食草动物,巨大的盲肠在腹内占据很大空间,几乎占据腹部四个象限,盲肠呈紫蓝色,直径约 4 cm,长约 40 cm。盲肠的盲端为阑尾,长约 10 cm。阑尾呈漏斗状,基部直径

1.5 cm,尖端约 1 cm。阑尾血供来源于回盲动脉(图2),因此处理阑尾血管时,应尽可能贴阑尾进行,防止损伤动脉主干,保证回肠血供。术中沿盲肠找阑尾是寻找阑尾的方法之一。

6. 盲肠近端与结肠和回肠(回盲部)相延续,结肠呈浅粉红色,宽约 1.5~2 cm。结肠往远端肠腔渐变细、粪便渐变硬,并呈卵圆形。与人不同,兔的结肠不分升、横、降、乙等部,无结肠带,也无脂肪垂,全部结肠皆有肠系膜,但均较短,因此有一定游离度。结肠与直肠相续。

7. 寻找脾脏之方法:如系左中、上腹切口,开腹后即可见到脾脏。如系右侧切口,将大网膜提起后轻轻向右下牵拉,即可将脾脏牵出切口;脾上极较固定,常不易完全牵至切口外。

8. 胃的分部和血供与人体基本相似,但胃右动脉在胃小弯角处进入胃(图3,图4),胃切除时应将其切断。

9. 胸膜反折线位于剑突中部之平面,故上腹手术切口之上限不可超过此平面,否则会切开胸膜,导致开放性气胸。

10. 术前未排尿者,膨胀的膀胱可上升至下腹上中 1/3 交界处,甚至达脐平面。一般应避免选用下腹部切口。

Appendix 3   Anesthesia Records, Operative Note and Postoperative Note

Anesthetic record, operative note and post-operative note are essential components of medical documentation and play important role in court or clinical trials. Poor medical records can jeopardise patient care and prejudice medicolegal cases. After an operative procedure on animal model, it is imperative for the anesthetist to complete the anesthetic record, and for the surgeon to immediately dictate the findings and key components of the case in an accurate and concise manner. Accurate record keeping is an important skill that should be mastered by all physicians and biomedical researchers.

It is important to provide accurate and detailed documentation of the location and severity of disease seen, in a scientific and realistic way. Therefore, each dictation should include any aspects of the surgery that were particularly difficult. Unnecessary details, and carelessness or falsification should be avoided. These surgical documentations are kept in the Department of Surgery for evaluation.

A. Anesthesia Records

1. Fill all blank spaces, including the identity information of the patient.

2. Document the date and time (24 hour clock): Five minutes past two o'clock and twenty minutes past six o'clock is noted in the following manner: 2:05 and 6:20, respectively. Total spent time of four hours and fifteen minutes may be noted as 4°15′.

3. Rate of pulse and respiration, and blood pressure are recorded on the anesthetic record chart using the symbols on the left side of **Animal Anesthesia Record**. These symbols are connected to form several curves according to the time.

4. Start of anesthesia or procedure, and end of anesthesia or procedure are recorded on bottom line of the anesthetic record chart using the symbols on the left side of **Animal Anesthesia Record**.

5. Each horizontal small box represents 10 minutes. The times are written on the top line as 9:00, 9:30, 10:00 and 10:30.

6. Except for anesthetic drugs, all drugs, fluids and blood products administered intraoperatively, including the name, dose and route, should be noted below the "Intra-Anesthetic Drugs".

7. Other related monitoring and support during the procedure and anesthetic recovery should be written under the "REMARKS".

8. Finally sign your name.

Animal Anesthesia Record

Grade _____　　Class _____
Group _____

Species _____　Fur Color _____　Sex _____　Weight _____ (kg)

Date _____　Animal No. _____

Preop. Dx. _____　Op. Planned _____

Postop. Dx _____　Op. Performed _____

Surgeon _____　1st Assist. _____　2nd Assist. _____　Scrub _____

Anesthetist _____　Circulator _____

Start Proc. _____　End Surgery _____　Total _____　Hr. (s) _____　Min. (s)

Start Anes. _____　End Anes. _____　Total _____　Hr. (s) _____　Min. (s)

Anesthesia _____　Anesthetic Drug, Dose & Route _____

	TIME		Pre-Anesthetic Drugs

● — ● Pulse
○ — ○ Resp.
∨ — ∨ Systo. B. P.
∧ — ∧ Diasto. B. P.
× — × Start & End of Anesth
⊙ — ⊙ Start & End of Surgery

200 180 160 140 120 100 80 60 40 20

Intra-Anesthetic Drugs

REMARKS

B. Operative note

1. Fill all blank spaces **in Animal Operative Record**, including patient demographics.

2. This is a note that is written right after the surgery, usually while in the operating or recovery room. The way to write down the time of procedure or anesthesia is described.

3. The key components of operative notes should include basic information, such as:

(1) Note type of anaesthesia (general or local) and the patient's positioning.

(2) State the details of the patient's preparation, including the name and concentration of the disinfectant, draping and catheterization.

163

Animal Operative Record

Grade _____ Class _____ Group _____

Species _____ Fur Color _____ Sex _____ Weight _____ (kg)

Date _____ Animal No. _____

Preop. Dx. _____ Op. Planned _____

Postop. Dx _____ Op. Performed _____

Surgeon _____ 1st Assist. _____ 2nd Assist. _____ Scrub _____

Anesthetist _____ Circulator _____

Start Proc. _____ End Surgery _____ Total _____ Hr. (s) _____ Min. (s)

Start Anes. _____ End Anes. _____ Total _____ Hr. (s) _____ Min. (s)

Anesthesia _____ Anesthetic Drug, Dose & Route _____

Findings:

Procedure(s) Performed & Description:

(3) Incision position, type (for example, midline), length and the situation in the layers of abdominal wall.

(4) Findings when entering the abdominal cavity: This should include fluid (ascites or pus) and gases and its volume and odor.

(5) Note the pathology discovered during the operation and other unexpected findings, such as anatomical variations, or accident.

(6) A step by step documentation of the operation should be noted, including major structures preserved, techniques used, intraoperative radiological images and microbiological specimens taken.

(7) Diagrams are useful especially in complex operations. Finally, include the type, size, and serial numbers of prosthesis and sutures used.

(8) Inspect the bleeding points and foreign body and drain the abdomen before closing abdominal wall.

(9) Estimated blood loss and type, note volume of fluid (blood) replacement and document tissue removed (specimen(s)) and the gross anatomy. Anything sent to pathology should be noted.

(10) Sign your name and write the date.

C. Postoperative note

1. Fill all blank spaces **in Animal Post-Operative Note**, including the identifying data of the patient.

2. Postoperative note should be carried out day by day and include ① subjective condition and mental status, and pain control; ② vital signs such as temperature, blood pressure, pulse and respirations; ③ physical exam: Chest and lungs; inspection of wound and surgical dressings; conditions of drains; characteristics and volume of output of drains; ④ impression and ⑤ plan. Document the date and time as following manner: 2012-04-15 or 2012-04-15-16:25.

3. The first Post operative note should be written immediately after the patient is sent back to ward and gives a brief description of the name of the procedure, vital signs during the procedure, anesthesia and it recovery, and then postoperative recovery.

4. At the first day (the day after the date of surgery), beside of subjective condition and mental status, the postoperative note should include appetite or nausea and vomitting, urination and defecation or passage of flatus by anus, wound and so on. A special attention should be paid to the special medical problems in surgical patients and the complications resulting from anesthesia and surgery, such as fever or fistula.

5. Time for suture removal is 7 days for abdomen incision. Suture removal and the situation of wound healing should be noted.

Animal Post-Operative Note

Grade _____ Class _____ Group _____

Species _____ Fur Color _____ Sex _____ Weight _____ (kg)

Animal # _____

Procedure(s)_____ Date _____

Findings:

In mainland of China, surgical wound is classified to three classes according to contamination: ①Class I/Clean: An uninfected operative wound in which no inflammation is encountered. In addition, clean wounds are primarily closed, such as the incisional wounds following thyroid surgery or hernia repair. ②Class II/Possible-Contaminated: An operative wound in which the respiratory, alimentary, genital, or urinary tracts are entered (e. g. gastrectomy), provided the wounds are primarily closed. Incision at the site where well preparation is limited, accidental wound treated by primary closure within 6 hours of injury and a newly closed wound which need to open again are included in this category. ③Class III/Contaminated: Wounds exposure to infected site or tissue, such as appendectomy following ruptured appendicitis or enterectomy following strangulated intestinal obstruction.

Surgical wound healing is also classified to three classes: ①Class A: The wound heals well and can be noted as "A". ②Class B: The wound heals with defect such as local erythema, painful induration, hematoma or seroma, but without purulence. It is noted as "B". ③Class C: The wound is infected and purulent, and needs re-opening and draining. It is noted as "C". As an instance, a well healing wound after excision of adenoma of thyroid or splenectomy can be noted as "I/A"; a wound with local erythema or hematoma after enterectomy may be noted as "II/B"; and an infected wound after peritonitis can be noted as "III/C", which needs suture removal, draining and secondary intention healing is expected.

Since 1990s, an wound classification system develops and is internationally accepted, in which wounds are classified to four types according to contamination: ①Clean: An uninfected operative wound in which no inflammation is encountered and the respiratory, alimentary, genital, or uninfected urinary tract is not entered. In addition, clean wounds are primarily closed and, if necessary, drained with closed drainage. Operative incisional wounds that follow nonpenetrating (blunt) trauma should be included in this category if they meet the criteria. ②Clean-Contaminated: An operative wound in which the respiratory, alimentary, genital, or urinary tracts are entered under controlled conditions and without unusual contamination. Specifically, operations involving the biliary tract, appendix, vagina, and oropharynx are included in this category, provided no evidence of infection or major break in technique is encountered. ③Contaminated: Open, fresh, accidental wounds. In addition, operations with major breaks in sterile technique (e. g. , open cardiac massage) or gross spillage from the gastrointestinal tract, and incisions in which acute, nonpurulent inflammation is encountered are included in this category. ④Dirty-Infected: Old traumatic wounds with retained devitalized tissue and those that involve existing clinical infection or perforated viscera. This definition suggests that the organisms causing postoperative infection were present in the operative field before the operation.

6. If the animal is dead intraoperatively or postoperatively, autopsy needs to be carried out to verify the cause of death. The death note should include:

(1) Have a concise review of the operative and postoperative course.

(2) Findings from autopsy.

(3) Cause of death is analyzed.

(4) Give a comment on experience and lesson.

附录三　动物手术麻醉记录、动物手术记录和动物手术术后观察记录的记录方法

　　麻醉记录、手术记录和术后观察(病程)记录是医疗文件(病历)的重要组成部分,也是科研资料累积的一环。不合格的医疗文件会导致误诊误治,给病人带来伤害,也不能为法庭提供真实的材料。动物手术实习后麻醉医生应该完成麻醉记录,手术者应该立即正确简明地记录手术所见,为临床工作打基础,同时也是科研工作方法的一种训练,应予重视。

　　上述记录的填写,必须有严格的科学态度和实事求是的精神,按照实际情况,认真细致、准确无误地逐项记录和填写,尤其要注意记录手术中的特殊发现、意外情况及其处理方法,不应草率从事,更不得弄虚作假。上述记录填写后交教研室计分存档。

一、麻醉记录

　　1. **动物手术麻醉记录**楣栏应逐项填写。

　　2. 手术及麻醉时间以下式记录:2点05分、6点20分,可分别写为2;05、6;20。手术耗时如为4小时15分,可简写为4°15′。

　　3. 脉搏、呼吸、血压分别以**动物手术麻醉记录**左侧的符号,按照相应的时间点记录,并将点连接成曲线。

　　4. 麻醉、手术的开始与终了,以**动物手术麻醉记录**左侧之符号,按照相应时间记录于表格底线上。

　　5. 小方格表,横行由左向右,每一小格代表10分钟,从记录开始时在最上方时间栏内记录时间,如9;00、9;30、10;00、10;30等。

　　6. 麻醉中用药项内记录术中应用的药品名称、剂量、方法和时间(不包括麻醉药物本身),包括输液(血)的种类、用量等。

　　7. 其他有关情况,如麻醉及手术过程中的主要情况或变化,麻醉苏醒情况等,均记录在**附记**栏内。

　　8. 最后由记录者(一般即麻醉师)签名。

二、手术记录

　　1. **动物手术记录**楣栏逐项填写。

　　2. 手术记录应该在手术后及时书写。时间记录方式同前。

　　3. 手术所见和手术经过包括以下各项:

　　(1) 麻醉方式和手术体位。

　　(2) 术野消毒情况,包括消毒药品名称、浓度及铺单情况等。

动物手术麻醉记录

_____年级　　　_____班次
_____小组

动物种类_____　毛色_____　　雌雄_____　体重_____（kg）

手术日期_____　　　动物编号_____

手术前诊断_____　　　拟施手术_____

手术后诊断_____　　　已施手术_____

手术者_____　第一助手_____　第二助手_____　手术护士_____

麻醉师_____　巡回护士_____

手术开始时间_____　终止时间_____　共_____时_____分

麻醉开始时间_____　终止时间_____　共_____时_____分

麻醉方法_____　麻醉药物品名、浓度和用量_____

（3）切口部位、切口种类、长度、开腹时腹腔各层组织的主要情况。

（4）切开腹膜后，腹腔内有无腹水、脓液、气体、气味及其量等，大网膜情况，术野中所见脏器情况，探查所见及触摸情况。

（5）寻找病变或所需脏器的情况和大体病理改变。是否发现异常情况，有无遇到困难或意外。

（6）有关脏器手术方法与步骤，如：主要脏器保留的方法，术中摄片，留取细菌性标本。记录组织切除和体液（血液）丢失情况。

动物手术记录

年级_____　班次_____　小组_____

动物种类_____　毛色_____　雌雄_____　体重_____（kg）

手术日期_____　动物编号_____

手术前诊断_____　拟施手术_____

手术后诊断_____　已施手术_____

手术者_____　第一助手_____　第二助手_____　手术护士_____

麻醉师_____　巡回护士_____

手术开始时间_____　终止时间_____　共_____时_____分

麻醉开始时间_____　终止时间_____　共_____时_____分

麻醉方法_____　麻醉药物品名、浓度和用量_____

手术方法和经过：

（7）复杂手术最好要绘图示意。注明植入假体的种类、大小和系列号以及缝线。

（8）手术结束关腹前，检查出血、异物存留等情况，放置引流。

（9）麻醉及病人耐受情况，出血量之估计，输血、输液情况。切取之标本记录肉眼所见，送病理检查。

（10）最后由手术者签名，并填写记录日期。

三、手术后观察记录

1. **术后记录楣栏逐项填写。**

2. 术后记录可以日记形式逐日记录，其内容应包括：①病人主观感觉和精神状态，以及疼痛情况；②生命体征，如：T、P、R、BP；③体格检查：心肺、创口、敷料、引流管情况（是否通畅、色和量）；④诊断；⑤处理计划。日期可简写成 2012-04-15。必要时加上记录时间，如 2012-04-15-16：25。

3. 第一次术后记录应该在手术当天记录，应包括手术名称、术中情况是否平稳、麻醉及恢复情况等，先简要加以描述，然后再记录术后情况。

4. 术后第一天（一般指手术之次日）以后，除记录一般情况（包括精神状态和活动能力等）外，每天记录的内容主要为：有无恶心呕吐、大小便或肛门排气情况、饮食情况、伤口情况，重点记录术前存在的内科夹杂症的变化，以及麻醉并发症和手术并发症的相关表现（如发热、瘘）。

5. 腹部手术一般于术后第七天拆线，应记录拆线及伤口（又称切口）愈合情况。

国内教科书一般按污染的程度将切口分为三类：①清洁切口（Ⅰ类切口），指一期缝合的无污染切口，如甲状腺手术切口、疝修补手术切口。②可能污染切口（Ⅱ类切口），指手术进入到呼吸道、消化道和泌尿生殖道,可能有污染的缝合切口,如胃切除手术。皮肤表面的细菌不容易被彻底消毒的部位,6 小时内经过清创术缝合的伤口、新缝合的切口再度切开者,都归此类。③污染切口(Ⅲ类切口),指直接暴露于感染区或组织的切口,如阑尾穿孔的阑尾切除术、肠梗阻肠坏死的手术。

切口愈合也分三级:①甲级愈合,用"甲"字代表,指伤口愈合优良,无不良反应。②乙级愈合,用"乙"字代表,指愈合缺陷,如红肿、硬结、血肿、积液,但未化脓。③丙级愈合,用"丙"字代表,指切口化脓,需要作切开引流处理。例如,甲状腺腺瘤切除术、脾切除术切口愈合优良,记录为Ⅰ/甲;小肠部分切除术后切口有红肿或血肿,记录为Ⅱ/乙;腹膜炎手术后腹壁切口化脓,需拆除缝线引流后二期愈合者,记录为Ⅲ/丙。

20 世纪 90 年代后,国际上趋向于按污染程度将切口分为四类:①清洁切口:见于无污染的经过皮肤消毒后的择期手术,未进入呼吸道、消化道或泌尿生殖道。由于感染率低,切口一期缝合;需要引流者,其引流为闭式引流;钝器伤后的手术切口只要符合上述标准也归入此类。②清洁—污染切口:手术中需要切开呼吸道、消化道或泌尿生殖道,创口得到保护,内容物无明显外溢。此外,涉及胆道、阑尾、阴道或咽部的手术,只要不存在感染依据,无菌术没有明显的漏洞(失误),也应该归入该类。③污染切口:是指新鲜的开放性创口。此外,无菌术有明显漏洞(失误)的手术(如:开胸心脏按压)、术中有明显大量胃肠内容物外溢的创口以及急性非化脓性炎症区域的切口都应该归入该类。④脏切口或污秽切口:其定义是在手术前引起术后感染的病原微生物已经存在于手术野,例如:有失活组织的陈旧创伤创口,先前就有临床感染或内脏穿孔的手术创口。

6. 动物手术中或术后死亡,酌情进行尸体解剖并填写死亡记录(可利用动物手术术后观察记录单记录)。其内容包括:

(1)将手术经过和术后情况,作一简单回顾性描述。

(2)尸体解剖发现之情况。

(3)死亡原因分析。

(4)经验和教训。

动物手术术后观察记录

年级_____ 班次_____ 小组_____

动物种类_____毛色_____雌雄_____体重_____(kg)

动物编号_____

手术名称_____ 手术日期_____

术后情况观察:

Appendix 4   An Example of Animal Operative Note

Animal Operative Record

Grade _____ **Class** _____ **Group** _____

Species dog **Fur Color** yellow **Sex** female **Weight** 17 (kg)

Date 2012−06−20 **Animal No.** _____

Preop. Dx. _____ **Op. Planned** enterectomy and end-to-end anastomosis

Postop. Dx. _____ **Op. Performed** as above

Surgeon Gang Wang **1st Assist.** Xiao-ming Li **2nd Assist.** Jie Wang **Scrub** Yan Zhang

Anesthetist Ping Zhou **Circulator** Xiao-ling Chen

Start Proc. 14:00 **End Surgery** 16:30 **Total** 2 **Hr.(s)** 30 **Min.(s)**

Start Anes. 13:40 **End Anes.** 16:30 **Total** 2 **Hr.(s)** 50 **Min.(s)**

Anesthesia general **Anesthetic Drug, Dose & Route** 2.5% thiopental 17 ml, iv

Findings, Procedure(s) Performed & Description:

With general anesthesia, the dog is stretched out on its back with its hocks tied to the corner cleats. The abdomen is clipped and the skin cleaned with detergent.

Skin preparation starts with twice application of alcoholic iodine at 3 percent followed by thrice with alcohol at 75 percent to remove iodine. Thereafter, surgical field is squared off and draped.

A 20-cm right upper abdominal midrectus (rectus-splitting) is used. When the skin and subcutaneous tissues are incised, hemostasis in the skin and subcutaneous tissues is achieved by hemostatic clamps. The wound is then protected from contamination by placing two towels secured by Allis clamps. The anterior rectus sheath is next incised in the line of the incision and the rectus is splitted to expose posterior rectus sheath. The posterior fascia of the rectus muscle is grasped with peritoneum and incised at a point of halfway, and the abdominal cavity is entered.

The peritoneal cavity is exposed by retractors and the exploration demonstrates that there are a few of milliliters of pink fluid with foul smelling, some small bowel and omentum are adhered to previous epigastric midline incision and the rest of the bowel looks normal, the spleen has been resected and the liver seems normal. An enterectomy is decided to carry out.

A segment of small bowel is delivered to the wound and its vascularization is inspected. When a segment of small bowel (about 10 cm) is selected to be resected, both sides of visceral peritoneum of related mesentery is divided with scissors in a wedge fashion and the straight vessels are serially clamped and divided between artery forceps, and complete hemostasis is secured by means of suture ligatures of 1/0 silk and a suture ligature at the proximal end. The demarcation of blood supply on the bowel is inspected. Either end of the small bowel segment to be cut is placed a Kocher clamp at an angle of 45° to longitudinal axis of the small bowel (longer bowel at mesenteric side is preserved). Two noncrushing intestinal clamps are then applied 5 cm away from each Kocher clamp, respectively. The surgical field is isolated with large square packs, the margins of the abdominal incision being covered with protective gauze to guard against contamination. The gut is divided close to the outside of Kocher clamp with a cautery (or knife). The segment containing the devascularized bowel is removed, and intestinal contents are removed by suction or by mopping with small swabs. The proximal and distal segments to be united are held together, and two seromuscular stay sutures (1/0 silk) were placed through both segments on the mesenteric and antimesenteric borders, respectively, to stabilize the position of the segments relative to each other. The posterior row of sutures, consisting of a continuous lock-stitch of 1/0 silk is introduced through all the layers. This suture is continued anteriorly as a Connell suture. Then, the two ends of the thread meet each other and are tied with the knot inside the intestinal lumen. The two intestinal clamps are unlocked and removed. The anterior and posterior seromuscular sutures are applied using interrupted sutures of 1/0 silk at intervals of 6 mm. The ends of the silk thread are cut short leaving approximately 3 mm from the knot. The patency of the stroma is proved and the defect in the mesentery is closed with interrupted silk sutures.

Inspect once more for possible bleeding point and foreign bodies in the abdomen. Count sponges and instruments. Omentum is interposed between the jejunum and body wall. The abdominal wall is closed without draining.

The course of the procedure is smooth. The blood loss is estimated about 50 ml. At the completion of the procedure, the dog was still unconscious, but the respiration was recovered, and sent back to the kennel.

The resected segment of bowel is not sent to pathology.

Gang Wang

2012-06-20

附录四　动物手术记录实例

动物手术记录

年级 _____ 班次 _____ 小组 _____

动物种类 ___狗___ 毛色 ___黄___ 雌雄 ___雌___ 体重 ___17___（kg）

手术日期 ___2012-06-20___ 动物编号 _____

手术前诊断 _____ 拟施手术 ___小肠部分切除端对端吻合术___

手术后诊断 _____ 已施手术 ___同上___

手术者 ___王钢___ 第一助手 ___李小明___ 第二助手 ___王洁___ 手术护士 ___张燕___

麻醉师 ___周平___ 巡回护士 ___陈晓玲___

手术开始时间 ___14:00___ 终止时间 ___16:30___ 共 _2_ 时 _30_ 分

麻醉开始时间 ___13:40___ 终止时间 ___16:30___ 共 _2_ 时 _50_ 分

麻醉方法 ___全麻___ 麻醉药物品名、浓度和用量 ___2.5％硫妥钠 17 ml iv___

手术方法和经过：

　　全麻成功后将狗平卧固定于手术台。腹部剪去毛发，用肥皂清洗。

　　用 3％碘酊消毒 2 遍，75％酒精脱碘，然后铺无菌巾和剖腹单。

　　取右中腹部经腹直肌切口，长约 20 cm，切开皮肤、皮下，结扎皮下出血点。护肤巾保护皮肤。切开腹直肌前鞘，纯性分离腹直肌，交替钳夹腹直肌后鞘和腹膜，确认避开腹内脏器或腹内网膜后，打开腹腔。

　　探查见腹腔内少许淡红色渗液，有恶臭味，肠管和网膜与原切口间有粘连，其余肠管无明显充血水肿，脾脏已切除，肝脏正常。决定行小肠部分切除。

　　取出一段小肠，观察小肠襻系膜的血管弓。选取拟切除的肠襻 10 cm，楔形剪开相应肠系膜两侧的腹膜层，分离肠系膜上的直血管，逐一分离、切断，近断端用"1"丝线结扎，并缝扎一道，观察肠襻缺血情况，在缺血肠管两端的正常肠管处与肠管纵轴呈 45°角（多留系膜缘，少留对系膜缘）各夹一把 Kocher 钳，然后在两把 Kocher 钳外侧 5 cm 各夹一把肠钳，用纱布保护，然后紧贴 Kocher 钳外缘切断肠管，用碘酊、酒精、生理盐水依次涂擦肠腔。在肠管的系膜缘及对系膜缘分别用"1"号丝线行浆肌层缝合作为牵引，用"1"号丝线在肠管的后壁从牵引线的一端开始做后壁全层连续锁边缝合，前壁连续全层内翻缝合（Connell 缝合）。松开并移去肠钳。然后行前、后壁浆肌层间断缝合，针距约 0.6 cm。剪断缝线，用拇指和食指检查吻合口能通过一食指尖。间断缝合肠系膜。

　　检查无活动性出血,清点纱布、器械和缝针无误,腹内未放引流。将大网膜放在肠管与腹壁之间。腹膜及腹直肌后鞘用"4"号丝线连续缝合,腹直肌前鞘用"1"号丝线间断缝合,然后用"1"号丝线间断缝合皮下及皮肤,切口涂龙胆紫。

　　手术顺利,麻醉满意,术中出血约 50 ml,术后全麻未醒,但呼吸已经恢复,送入狗房。

　　切下的肠管未送病检。

记录:王钢

2012-06-20

Appendix 5　Minor Surgical Techniques

A. Insertion of indwelling（Foley）urinary catheter

（A）Personnel Required

One person can insert an indwelling urinary catheter unaided. A chaperone is advisable if male medical personnel are catheterizing a woman. An assistant is helpful if the patient is uncooperative.

（B）Equipment & Supplies Required

A Foley insertion tray that contains the items listed below：①Foley catheter of the appropriate size and a sample tube for obtaining a sterile urine specimen. The Foley catheter consists of a double-lumen rubber tube with a terminal retaining balloon（Fig 1, Fig. 2）. ②Sterile gloves, towels and a fenestrated drape. ③Urinary drainage bag and connecting tube. ④Sterile lubricant. ⑤Antiseptic solution and sterile cotton balls. ⑥Sterile syringe, 5-to 10-ml, filled with enough sterile water. In addition, adhesive tape, alcohol burner and match should be supplied if conical-tip or Robingson urethral catheter without a terminal retaining balloon is used.

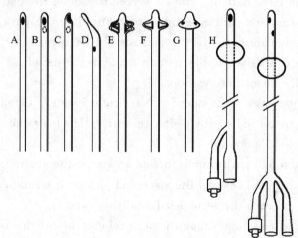

Fig. 1　Urinary catheters. A. Conical-tip urethral catheters. B. Robinson urethral catheter.
C. Whistle-tip urethral catheter. D. Coudé hollow olive-tip catheter. E. Malecot self-retaining, four-wing urethral catheter. F. Malecot self-retaining two-wing catheter. G. Pezzer self-retaining drain, open-end head, used for cystotomy drainage. H. Foley-type balloon catheter. I. Foley-type, three-way balloon catheter
图1　导尿管的种类

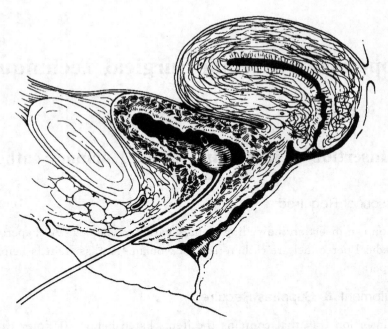

Fig. 2   Anatomical position of the Foley catheter
图 2   Foley 导尿管在膀胱内的解剖示意图

（C）Procedure

1. Put on a cap and face mask. Wash your hands with soap and warm water. Take sterile kit with you and go to the patient. Explain the procedure to the patient and try to get a good cooperation from patient. Have a screen to isolate the patient.

2. Patient's trousers and pants are taken off. For the male patient, the supine position is ideal. For the female patient, the legs should be spread, or "frog-legged". The sterile kit may be placed between the patient's thighs; otherwise, work from a sterile Mayo setup specifically for catheterization.

3. Stand on the patient's right side if you are right handed. Open the antiseptic packet, and moisten the cotton balls provided with antiseptic (benzalkonium bromide at 0. 1 per cent, chlorhexidine or iodophors).

4. Pick up a cotton ball with thumb forceps to sterile the genitalia and perineal area in a circle and outward fashion. Discard the swab and pick up a second cotton ball and repeat the work once more. Discard the second ball and the forceps.

5. Put on sterile gloves, and drape the perineal area before making the second sterilization.

For male patient, grasp the penis at the shaft below the glans and retract foreskin (be sure to replace at end of procedure) with your nondominant hand. Using the dominant hand and forceps, pick up cotton ball soaked in antiseptic solution and cleanse the penis beginning at the meatus and working toward the base.

For female patient, part the labia with your nondominant hand and expose the urethral meatus. Using the dominant hand and forceps, pick up cotton ball soaked in antiseptic solution and cleanse perineal area. This should be done with a wiping motion anterior to posterior from the clitoris toward the anus. A new cotton ball should be used for each wiping motion.

6. Coat the tip of the catheter with lubricating jelly. It is often helpful to place some on the meatus as well. Put a single loop in the Foley catheter for easier handling, grasp the catheter about 5 cm from the tip in the right hand. Slowly insert catheter through meatus. Insert catheter approximately 5 cm in adult female patient or until urine is seen flowing out the end of the catheter, or 17.5~22.5 cm in an adult male patient.

7. Inflate the balloon with the appropriate amount of sterile water (usually 5 ml), and withdraw the catheter gently until the balloon is pulled snugly against the trigone (Fig 2).

8. Collect a small amount of urine in a sterile container for appropriate studies (a urinalysis should be obtained routinely), and then connect the catheter to the urinary drainage bag.

（D）Note

1. Strictly observe sterile technique. Sterile technique is essential, as 40% of all nosocomial infections are urinary tract infections.

2. The most common mistake in catheterization of the female bladder is to miss the urethral meatus and inadvertently slip the catheter into the vagina. No urine will return. Remove the catheter, which has now been contaminated by vaginal flora; obtain a new, sterile catheter; and try again.

3. The collection unit must be placed lower than the level of the bladder and drainage of urine occurs by gravity.

4. Insert and pull the catheter gently to avoid mucous membrane of urethra damage.

B.　Wound Dressing Change

The aim of wound dressing change is to create an environment enabling wound healing by cleansing the wound, draining the wound, and removal of foreign body from wound.

（A）Preparation

1. The room should be cleaned at least a half hour ahead before the dressing change.

2. Review the medical document and check the wound to estimate how many dressing materials, solutions or instruments are required.

3. Put on a cap and face mask. Wash your hands with soap or an antibacterial cleanser and warm water.

4. Equipment and Supplies Required: 2 sterile bowls (one for sterile items, the other for dirty dressing and trash), 2 thumb forceps, suture scissors, sterile gloves, some cotton balls soaking with alcohol or normal saline, gauze and draining material and adhesive tape.

(B) Procedure

1. Observe for drainage, and odor if any.

2. Removing the old dressing: Don gloves to protect yourself and avoid contact with bodily fluids. Start by picking up the strip of adhesive plaster and pull it towards the incision with the fingers of one hand. To ease discomfort, using the fingers of your free hand to gently push down the skin away from the adhesive (Fig. 3). Remove one side as far as the incision, then go to the other side and repeat the procedure. This avoids pulling on the wound which can cause pain. When the dressing must be changed frequently the adhesive in contact with the skin can be left in place or adhesive straps can be used (Fig. 4).

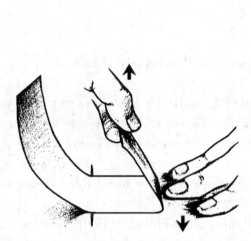

Fig. 3　Removing the strip of adhesive plaster
图 3　揭胶布的方法

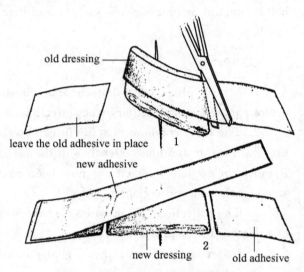

Fig. 4　Leave the old adhesive in place
图 4　与皮肤黏着紧密的胶布也可以不揭

The secondary dressing is removed by hand and the primary is by forceps. Carefully throw the old dressing into the bowl for dirty dressing.

The wound may have dried under the primary dressing, and it may be adhered. This tends to be the most painful procedure of the whole dressing change, and going slowly is important. Moistening the dressing using normal saline can often loosen the primary dressing from the wound bed and decreases the pain of dressing change.

3. Cleansing the wound: Place a towel under the wound to catch drainage. One forceps is used for picking up items from the bowl for sterile materials and passing to other forceps. The late forceps is allowed to contact wound. The periwound area is wiped from the wound edge outward using alcohol cotton ball. The wound is cleaned only with normal

saline. Normal saline is sufficient for removing excess bacteria while maintaining the natural healing processes at the base of the wound. Remove foreign body, suture knot, dead bone and devitalized tissue. Discard the soft cloth or piece of gauze into the dirty bowl.

4. Apply new dressing and secure with tape

(1) Applying the primary dressing: The primary dressing is chosen to keep the wound moist, but not too wet. Moist wounds healed more rapidly than those that were left exposed to the air or covered with traditional dry dressings. If the wound becomes too wet, this doesn't cause significant damage to the wound, but it is messier and can cause odor problems. Therefore, the primary dressing is chosen to keep a moist, clean wound bed. If the granulation tissue is healthy, cover with a low-adherent dressing such as petrolatum gauze.

(2) Applying the secondary dressing: The secondary dressing is chosen to fasten the primary dressing tightly to the body. This is to protect the wound from trauma and also to assist in any excessive drainage.

5. Edematous granulation tissue: The presence of edema often increases the volume of exudate produced by chronic wounds. Dressings and swabbing materials should be avoided that leave fibers in the wound bed as foreign bodies prolong the inflammatory response and delay healing. Chronic wound fluid differs from that of acute wounds and excess exudate has an adverse effect on wound healing. Edema control in the edematous limb can be obtained with compression bandaging, intermittent pneumatic compression or negative pressure devices.

6. Remove your gloves and take all of your trash out to your trash receptacle if possible. Wash your hands again!

(C) Note

1. A simple dressing change is a clean procedure, not a sterile one, unless your facility requires it to be. But the principles of asepsis or aseptic techniques should be rigorously followed. An infected wound should be opened and completely drained.

2. If there are several patients whose wound dressings need to be changed, the clean wound is changed first and the severe infected wound last.

3. Bed isolation should be carried out for the wounds of gas gangrene, tetanus and Pseudomonas aeruginosa. The dressings removed from these wound should be burned immediately and the instruments sterilized separately.

4. "I dress the wounds, God heals them", Paré said 400 years ago. He also suggested "treating wounds gently". Wound healing is natural processes. Chemicals have no benefit to wound healing. Do **NOT** use antiseptics such as hydrogen peroxide, alcohol, sodium hydrochlorite (Dakin solution) or iodine. These chemicals can damage sensitive tissue and prevent healing. Scientific studies have shown that these cleaning agents are very toxic to the body's natural processes for healing a wound and will wash away the biochemicals nee-

ded for wound repair. **As a rule of thumb，put nothing into a wound that you would not put in your eye.**

C. Suture Removal

（A）Preparation

The preparation for suture removal is the same as wound dressing change.

（B）Procedure

1. According to wound contamination classification，classify the wound as clean，possible-contaminated or contaminated.

2. Removing the old dressing and observe the wound and classify it according to surgical wound healing classification：①Class A：The wound heals well or primary intention healing. ②Class B：The wound heals with defect such as local erythema，painful induration，hematoma or wound edge ill-apposition. ③Class C：The wound is disrupted or infected with purulence.

3. Cleansing the wound：One forceps is used for picking up items from the bowl for sterile materials and passing to other forceps. The late forceps is allowed to contact wound.

Class A wound healing：①The wound area is gently wiped from the center of the wound outward using alcohol cotton ball. ②Pick up one end of the suture with thumb forceps，and cut as close to the skin as possible where the suture enters the skin. ③Gently pull the suture strand out through the side opposite the knot with the forceps (Fig. 2-40). To prevent risk of infection，the suture should be removed without pulling any portion that has been outside the skin back through the skin. Wiped the wound area once more using alcohol cotton ball.

Class B wound healing：After suture removal，the wound with local erythema and induration should be treated with physical therapy，hematoma or seroma should be drained，and ill-apposition wound be dressed.

Class C wound healing：The wound is drained for secondary intention wound healing.

4. Do not forget to write a note of the wound healing.

（C）Keep in mind that：

1. Sutures should be removed using aseptic and sterile technique.

2. When the wound has healed so that it no longer needs the support of non-absorbable suture material，skin sutures must be removed. The length of time the sutures remain in place depends upon the age of patient，the rate of healing and the nature of the wound. Sutures should be removed "before the epithelium has migrated into deeper parts of the

dermis. To prevent widening of the scar, the wound edges must be taped".

D. Internal jugular venous catheterization

（A）Indications

Internal jugular vein catheterization is performed to gain access to the central venous system for administration of fluids or measurement of central venous pressure.

（B）Personnel Required

The operator performing internal jugular vein catheterization requires an assistant to help handle sterile materials and position the patient.

（C）Equipment & Supplies Required

①Materials for skin sterilization. ②Lidocaine, 1%, with 10-ml syringe. ③Container of intravenous fluid with all necessary tubing. ④Prepackaged sterile venous cutdown trays including: insertion set an introducing needle and a 30 cm long radiopaque central venous catheter, drapes, gauze sponges （10×10 cm）, silk skin suture （size 000 or 0000） on a cutting needle, needle holder, straight scissors and syringe （2 ml for use as a probe）. Assemble and arrange all of the necessary equipment, including the container of intravenous fluid and intravenous tubing, and make sure the tubing has been flushed to remove air.

（D）Procedure

1. Put on a cap and face mask. Wash your hands with soap and warm water. Take sterile kit with you and go to the patient. Explain the procedure to the patient and try to get a good cooperation from patient.

2. Positioning of the Patient: Use a bed which has a movable headboard. The patient should be supine, with the head turned 45 degrees away from the side selected for insertion. Usually it is easier to position a catheter into the superior vena cava from the right internal jugular vein than from the left. Place the patient in a head down 15 degrees Trendelenburg position in order to fully distend the internal jugular vein and also to create increased pressure inside the vein, thus decreasing the chances of air embolism during insertion.

3. Put on sterile gloves and stand on the patient's cephalad.

4. Observe sterile technique and sterilize the skin around the area of insertion from the clavicle to the ear, and drape the patient.

5. The sternocleidomastoid muscle will be clearly outlined when the patient lifts the head slightly. Make a mental picture of the triangle formed by the 2 heads of the muscle, which has its apex pointed cephalad and its base formed by the clavicle. Palpate the carotid

artery, and make a mental note of the course of the internal jugular vein, which runs lateral and deep to the artery.

6. Choose a point near the apex of the triangle formed by the sternocleidomastoid, and anesthetize the skin with the 1% lidocaine.

7. Make a probe by placing a 22-gauge needle on the 2 ml syringe. Pierce the skin near the apex of the triangle formed by the sternocleidomastoid, and direct the needle at a 30 to 45 degree angle toward the ipsilateral nipple. The needle should pierce the vein after advancing 2.5~4 cm. If it does not, reposition the needle in the subcutaneous tissue, and probe more medially, always keeping the left index finger on the carotid artery for reference. Once the needle has entered the internal jugular vein, dark venous blood should flow freely into the syringe (Fig. 5).

Caution: Do not use the larger catheter insertion needle if the vein cannot be located with the probing needle.

8. Withdraw the probing needle. Now place the catheter insertion needle, and follow the course of the probing needle to enter the internal jugular vein. Always recheck the landmarks and position of the carotid artery while inserting this large needle. Once the needle has entered the vein, dark venous blood will flow freely into the syringe.

9. When it is clear that the needle is properly positioned in the lumen of the vein, disconnect the syringe, and immediately occlude the orifice of the catheter to prevent air embolization during inspiration. Pass the catheter through the needle into the vein.

10. When the catheter is fully inserted, check again to be sure that there is good return,

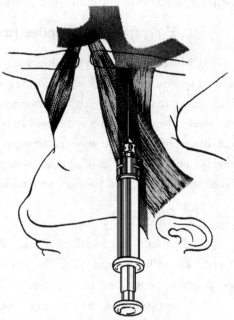

Fig. 5　Internal jugular vein
catheterization—anterior approach
图 5　颈内静脉穿刺置管（前路法）

attach the intravenous tubing, and start the fluid infusion. Anchor the catheter in place with fine silk skin suture. Make sure that the catheter is well secured, and tape it in place. Cover the insertion site with a sterile gauze pad.

E. Intraosseous infusion

Intraosseous infusion through cannulation of the medullary cavity in the anteromedial aspect of the tibia in an uninjured extremity is a safe and efficacious method for emergency vascular access in the infant and small child. The procedure is simple and, sadly, often overlooked when vascular access is a lifesaving imperative. Critical points are outlined in Fig. 6.

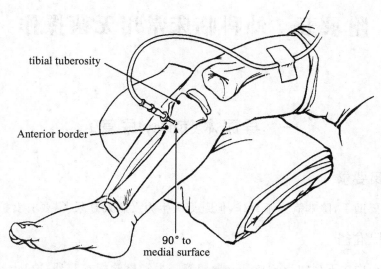

tibial tuberosity

Anterior border

90° to
medial surface

Fig. 6　Intraosseous infusion
图 6　婴幼儿骨髓腔输液(与内侧平面呈 90°进针)

1. Sterile technique is mandatory.

2. The anteromedial surface of the proximal tibia is the safest and most reliable site for placement.

附录五 外科临床常用无菌操作

一、导尿术（Foley 尿管）

（一）人员要求

导尿不需要助手，除非病人不合作，但是男医生为女病人导尿，需要有女护士陪伴。

（二）用品准备

无菌导尿包中含下列物品：①Foley 导尿管一根和检验标本容器，Foley 导尿管是一种头端带有水囊的双腔导尿管（图 1，图 2）；②无菌手套一副和治疗巾、手术洞巾；③储尿袋和连接管；④灭菌液状石蜡；⑤消毒液和棉球；⑥5～10 ml 注射器。如果用普通导尿管（头端不带水囊），还需备胶布、酒精灯及火柴。

（三）操作方法

1. 医生戴帽子和口罩，洗手。备齐用品，携至病人处，说明目的取得合作，并用屏风适当遮挡病人。

2. 病人仰卧，脱去裤管。男病人仰卧位，两腿屈膝自然分开即可；女病人两腿须屈曲外展呈"蛙式"。将导尿包放在病人的两腿之间，也可以放在导尿专用车上。

3. 右利者站在病人右侧。打开导尿包。用消毒液（0.1%苯扎溴铵、氯己定或碘伏）将棉球浸透。

4. 用无菌镊子夹消毒液棉球，进行外消毒。消毒以尿道口为中心，由内向外做环状擦洗消毒，换一个棉球再擦洗一次，消毒毕将镊子弃去。

5. 戴手套，铺洞巾，进行内消毒。

男病人：用左手捏住阴茎头下方的体部，将包皮推向后方（注意：导尿结束后应该将包皮恢复原位）显露尿道口；右手用无菌镊子夹消毒液棉球，以尿道口为中心进行消毒。擦洗两次。

女病人：用左手分开小阴唇，显露尿道口；右手用无菌镊子夹消毒液棉球，自前向后对尿道口进行擦洗消毒。每次换新棉球。

6. 尿管头部沾无菌液状石蜡，若在尿道口涂些无菌液状石蜡更好。把 Foley 导尿管弯一个圈抓在手中，手指捏住导尿管头部距尖端 5 cm 处，将导尿管轻轻插入尿道。女性成人插入深度约 5 cm，或见尿从尿管中自行流出，将尿流入碗内；男性成人插入深度约 20 cm 左右。

7. 水囊注水 5 ml,轻轻将尿管向外拉,使水囊位于膀胱三角区(图 2)。

8. 留取尿液进行尿常规检查。需留尿培养者,直接将尿导入试管,以防污染。然后,将导尿管与集尿袋连接。

(四) 注意事项

1. 严格执行无菌操作。这一点极为重要,40%医院内感染是尿路感染。

2. 女性导尿时常发生的错误是导尿管误插入阴道,此时应立即拔出,另更换一根无菌导尿管重插。

3. 集尿袋放置的位置应该比膀胱低,让尿液随重力流入尿袋。

4. 插入及拔出导尿管动作务必轻柔,切忌粗暴,以免损伤尿道黏膜。

二、创口敷料更换术(换药)

换药的目的是清洁伤口、保证创口引流通畅、去除创口内坏死组织和异物,使创口早日愈合。

(一) 换药前准备

1. 换药前半小时内不要扫地。

2. 复习病历,了解伤口情况,估计敷料用量以及器械和材料的准备。

3. 戴好帽子和口罩,用肥皂或消毒液以及温水洗手。

4. 器械和敷料准备:一般需要 2 个灭菌碗(一个放无菌物品,另一个供盛放脏敷料和废物);2 把镊子;线剪;无菌手套;酒精棉球及盐水棉球、纱布、引流条、胶布。

(二) 操作方法

1. 观察创口的引流,注意有无异味。盛脏敷料的碗距病人近些,盛灭菌敷料的碗距病人远些。

2. 揭去旧敷料:戴手套避免体液污染,先用手揭开胶布一端的角,向切口方向揭胶布,一直揭至切口处。为了减轻疼痛,揭胶布时可以用另一只手压住胶布旁的皮肤,按毛发生长方向自毛根向毛梢、尽可能贴皮肤揭下胶布(图 3)。然后,按同法揭胶布的另一端。用这种方法揭胶布可以减轻疼痛。如果需要频繁更换敷料,与皮肤黏着的胶布可以剪下留在原位,然后将新胶布贴在其上(图 4)。取下外层敷料,再用镊子取下内层敷料及引流物,放入脏敷料碗中。

内层敷料可能因为干结而与创面紧贴,因此,揭敷料可能是更换敷料最疼痛的环节,重要的是耐心。用生理盐水湿润内层敷料有助于干结敷料的揭去,同时减少疼痛。

3. 清洁伤口:在创口下方垫一块治疗巾,以免液体污染床褥或衣裤。一把镊子用作传递灭菌敷料,另一把镊子接触创面。先用酒精棉球轻拭创口周围皮肤(消毒范围约相当于敷料范围或略大,或距伤口 5 cm)后用无菌生理盐水棉球轻沾创口。生理盐水可以去除创口内的细菌,并且能维持创口从创底开始自然愈合。清除创口内的异物、线头、死骨及腐肉等。不得用擦洗过创口周围皮肤的棉球沾洗创面。严防将纱布、棉球遗留在伤口内。

4．盖新敷料,用胶布固定

(1) 内层敷料:要求内层敷料能保持创面湿润,但不要过湿。湿润的创面比暴露的创面愈合快,比传统干敷料覆盖的创面愈合快。创面过湿的害处并不大,但是敷料容易脏,出现气味。因此,要求内层敷料能维持湿润、干净的创面。一般无严重感染的健康肉芽伤口,可用低粘敷料覆盖,如凡士林纱布。

(2) 外层敷料:外层敷料的作用是将内层敷料固定于原位、保护创面免受损伤,还有吸湿作用。

5．水肿肉芽组织:创面水肿常伴有渗液,是慢性创口的特点。此时,要尽可能避免应用棉敷料或棉球,以免纤维遗留在创口内形成异物,不利于创口愈合。慢性创口渗液不同于急性创口渗液,它不利于创口愈合。四肢水肿创面的处理方法是加压包扎、间断气压治疗和局部负压吸引。

6．脱去手套,把所有脏物放入指定的脏物容器中。再次认真洗手!

(三) 注意事项

1．一般的创口敷料更换是一种清洁操作,并不是无菌操作,除非有特殊要求。但是,医生应该严格遵守无菌外科技术。

2．先换清洁的创口,再换感染轻微的,最后换感染严重的创口。感染创口应该敞开并引流。

3．气性坏疽、破伤风、绿脓杆菌等感染伤口,必须严格执行床边隔离制度,污染的敷料需及时焚毁,使用的器械应单独消毒灭菌。

4．400年前,Paré 就认为"我的任务是包扎伤口,伤口愈合是上帝的事",并提出"善待"伤口组织的概念。也就是说伤口的愈合完全是人体的本能,不依靠任何药物。**不要在伤口内用抗菌剂**,诸如:过氧化氢溶液、酒精、盐酸钠(Dakin 溶液)以及碘。研究表明,这些清洁剂不利于伤口愈合,并且会吸去伤口修复所必需的生化物质。一句话,**医生要像爱护眼睛一样爱护伤口的组织,就像你不会把任何刺激性东西放在眼睛里一样,请勿将任何药物或刺激性物品放在伤口内。**

三、拆　　线

(一) 拆线前准备

与敷料更换术相同,同时准备拆线剪刀1把。

(二) 操作方法

1．根据切口污染分类方案,明确切口分类,即:无菌切口、可能污染切口抑或污染切口。

2．取下切口敷料,正确判定愈合情况:①甲级:切口部位无不良反应的一期愈合。②乙级:愈合欠佳。可有缝线周围炎,红肿、硬结、血肿、积液或表面皮肤裂开等。③丙级:切口完全裂开或化脓。

3．清洁伤口:一把镊子用作传递无菌物品,一把镊子接触切口。

切口甲级愈合：①用酒精棉球从中央向外周轻拭切口；②用镊子提起缝线的一头，紧贴缝线的入皮处剪断；③轻轻将缝线的另一端拉出，紧贴皮肤剪断拆除缝线（图2-40）。为了防止感染，**抽线时勿使暴露于皮肤外面的缝线进入皮肤内**。拆线后再用酒精棉球将切口擦拭一遍。

切口乙级愈合：缝线周围炎及轻度红肿硬结的切口，拆除缝线后热敷即可；有血肿或积液者应引流，表面皮肤裂开可用蝶形胶布条拉拢切口。

切口丙级愈合：应拆线后充分引流或作二期缝合。

4. 记录切口愈合情况。

（三）注意事项

1. 严格遵守无菌外科技术，操作轻柔。

2. 切口已经愈合，不需要缝线支持时，不可吸收缝线应该拆除。不同组织、不同年龄、不同部位的切口愈合速度不一致。应试探切口的愈合强度，决定全部拆线或间断拆线，不可在伤口愈合不良时，贸然一次拆除全部缝线。

四、颈内静脉穿刺置管术

（一）适应证

急救或长期静脉输液或给药，周围静脉穿刺未获成功者；某些特殊检查，如右心导管检查术，测定中心静脉压。

（二）人员要求

做颈内静脉穿刺置管需要有一名助手帮助递无菌物品和为病人摆放体位。

（三）用品准备

①皮肤消毒用品；②1％利多卡因溶液和10 ml注射器；③输液和连接管；④包含下列物品的静脉切开包：置管装置（主要有导管针和30 cm长不透放射线的中心静脉导管各一枚）、手术单、纱布、丝线和三角针、持针器、线剪和用于试穿刺的2 ml注射器。所有器械和物品都安装好，处于备用状态，如：静脉输液管应该与输液瓶相接，输液管内的气泡已经驱除。

（四）操作方法

1. 备齐用品，携至病人处，说明目的以取得合作。

2. 病床的床头板应该能拆卸。病人仰卧，头向对侧转45°。一般来讲，右侧颈内静脉的穿刺比较容易成功。头低脚高位15°，使颈内静脉充盈，增加静脉内压力，减少气栓的风险。

3. 医生站在病人头侧，戴手套。

4. 按无菌规则对锁骨至耳部的区域进行常规皮肤消毒，以胸锁乳突肌中点（乳突与锁骨头的中点）为中心铺巾。

5. 让病人稍抬头，辨清胸锁乳突肌两头所构成的三角，该三角的尖指向头侧，三角的底边是锁骨。触到颈动脉,构画颈内静脉的走向。颈内静脉行走于颈动脉的外侧、深面。

6. 在三角尖端的上方用 1‰利多卡因进行局部浸润麻醉。

7. 用 2 ml 注射器接细针头进行试穿,左手食指和中指扣压颈动脉,紧贴动脉外侧、三角顶端的梢头侧穿刺进针。穿刺针与皮肤成 30～45°角,针头指向同侧乳头。一般进针 2.5～4 cm 即可穿到静脉。若第一次穿刺不成功,二次穿刺时,可以调整针头方向使之稍偏向内侧。穿刺时,左手食指不要离开颈动脉作为参照。一旦针头进入颈内静脉,暗红色静脉血即可涌入注射器(图 5)。

注意:不要一开始就用粗的导管针穿刺。

8. 退出试穿针,用导管针按试穿针的路径进行穿刺。粗针穿刺前,要重新确认解剖标志和触摸颈动脉。针头进入静脉后,可以见到暗红色血液涌入注射器。

9. 确定针头在位后,固定针头位置,移去注射器,立即用手指堵住针孔防止吸气时发生气栓,将导管插入静脉。

10. 导管插入后,再次检查回血是否正常,拔出导管针,连接输液管。用细丝线将导管与皮肤固定。用无菌纱布覆盖穿刺部位。

五、婴幼儿骨髓腔输液

在婴幼儿,在无损伤侧下肢的胫骨前内侧置管进行骨髓腔输液是一种紧急建立血管通道的手段,且安全有效。遗憾的是,在病儿需要紧急建立静脉通道时,这一途径常常被遗忘。建立骨髓腔输液通道的要点见图 6。

1. 必须重视无菌操作。

2. 胫骨近端的前内侧平面是置管最常用的部位,也是最安全、最可靠的部位。